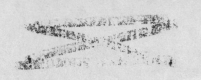

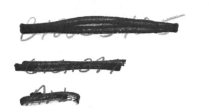

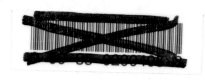

THE QUEEN OF FATS

CALIFORNIA STUDIES IN FOOD AND CULTURE

DARRA GOLDSTEIN, EDITOR

THE QUEEN OF FATS

WHY OMEGA-3s WERE REMOVED FROM THE WESTERN DIET AND WHAT WE CAN DO TO REPLACE THEM

SUSAN ALLPORT

UNIVERSITY OF CALIFORNIA PRESS
BERKELEY   LOS ANGELES   LONDON

University of California Press, one of the most distinguished
university presses in the United States, enriches lives around
the world by advancing scholarship in the humanities, social
sciences, and natural sciences. Its activities are supported by
the UC Press Foundation and by philanthropic contributions
from individuals and institutions. For more information, visit
www.ucpress.edu.

University of California Press
Berkeley and Los Angeles, California

University of California Press, Ltd.
London, England

Library of Congress Cataloging-in-Publication Data

Allport, Susan.
    The queen of fats : why omega-3s were removed from the
Western diet and what we can do to replace them / Susan Allport.
        p.   cm. — (California studies in food and culture ; 15)
    Includes bibliographical references and index.
    ISBN-13, 978-0-520-24282-1 (alk. paper),
    ISBN-10, 0-520-24282-3 (alk. paper)
    1. Essential fatty acids in human nutrition.   2. Omega-3
fatty acids—Health aspects.   3. Omega-3 fatty acids—
Research—History. I. Title. II. Series.
QP752.O44A45   2006
612.3′97—dc22   2005035605

Manufactured in the United States of America

15   14   13   12   11   10   09   08   07
10   9   8   7   6   5   4   3   2

This book is printed on New Leaf EcoBook 60, containing
60% post-consumer waste, processed chlorine free; 30% de-
inked recycled fiber, elemental chlorine free; and 10% FSC-
certified virgin fiber, totally chlorine free. EcoBook 60 is acid-
free and meets the minimum requirements of ANSI/ASTM
D5634–01 (Permanence of Paper).

FOR THE SCIENTISTS WHO PIECED TOGETHER THIS STORY
AND FOR MY FAMILY, THE MOST NOURISHING A WRITER COULD HAVE

CONTENTS

ONE

WHAT'S FOR DINNER?

I look upon it, that he who does not mind
his belly will hardly mind anything else.

SAMUEL JOHNSON, 1763

THE YEAR 2003 WILL BE REMEMBERED AS A TIME WHEN AMERICA LOST
its dietary senses. Overnight, it seemed, this country switched
from a low-fat regime, in which people shunned every form of
visible fat, to the Atkins regime, in which fat consumption was
encouraged but carbohydrates were to be avoided. Jack Sprat,
who could eat no fat, suddenly became Sprat's wife and could eat
no lean.

The accumulated nutritional advice from decades of research
was tossed aside like an old blanket, and grocery stores were suddenly filled with such gastronomical oxymora as low-carb bread
and beer. Thin women in tight jeans were overheard saying that
they loved beets and apples but had to stay away from them
because of all their carbs. Large men in business suits ordered
bunless burgers dripping with bacon grease and raved about their
diets. Anyone coming back to the United States after time spent
in Europe or Asia had an Alice-in-Wonderland experience, as
several returnees told me: black had become white and carbohydrates, the food that feeds most of the world's peoples, including
the world's leanest peoples, were suddenly the bad guys.

But 2003 should be remembered not only as the year that America lost its dietary senses (which it did) but also as the year that the center would no longer hold. By 2003, the nutritional advice given out to Americans by government agencies like the United States Department of Agriculture and medical organizations like the American Heart Association had become so out of sync with current research and biological understanding that schisms and confusion became inevitable.

It is unfortunate that those schisms took the form of total rejection, on the part of many Americans, of all the acquired wisdom about what constitutes a healthy diet. But that's what happens when the center doesn't hold, when the marketplace is full of such absurdities as overly sweetened breakfast cereals, such as Cocoa Puffs and Lucky Charms, being endorsed by the American Heart Association (because they have no cholesterol or saturated fat)—when the oversimplistic, low-fat mantra of the 1980s and 1990s made the Atkins craze almost inescapable. As a dieter in Texas confides, "Eating low-fat guarantees that I will binge on fried foods. Eating low-carb guarantees that I will binge on a bag of chips."

Much of the country is now on that fried-food, high-fat binge (or has binged out on Atkins and moved on). Many of us are more confused than ever about the simplest, most fundamental of questions: What should we have for dinner?

In the midst of this confusion, I'd like to throw my hat into the ring of nutritional advice with a tribute to one food, or family of foods: the fatty acids popularly known as the omega-3s. Because these fats were not recognized as being essential to human health until the 1980s, most current recommendations and nutritional advice took shape without them. At the same time, they were being eliminated from many foods because their presence caused problems with product stability and shelf life. Their absence, from our foods and our guidelines, is a key, a large and growing number of scientists believe, to many of our health problems—and even our befuddlement about food.

I have none of the usual qualifications to write this homage. I am neither a physician who treats the diseases to which people who are deficient in these fats are prone nor a scientist who has spent a lifetime researching the membranes that these fats call home. But that may be an advantage, since scientists and physicians tend to focus on the one piece of the puzzle they are looking at and these fats, as it turns out, affect the entire body in many different ways.

Rather, I am a science writer, a curious denizen of twenty-first-century America with a long-standing interest in food and the difficulties of being a human omnivore, and I will try to present the big picture. Quite simply, trying to understand health and diet without an appreciation of these fats is like trying to understand earthquakes without knowledge of plate tectonics, or motion without knowledge of physics. Until we revise our foods and guidelines to incorporate all that has been learned about omega-3 fatty acids in the past fifty years, our diet will be lacking in a very important way.

After I introduce these fats, I think you will begin to see why they deserve this book of their own. This introduction will involve some chemistry, but only what is necessary and most of which will be familiar to cooks, shoppers, and nutrition-conscious readers. Further explanations and diagrams can be found in the glossary, which begins on page 159. All that readers need to know from the get-go is that fatty acids, the components of fats and cell membranes, are chains of carbons and hydrogens with an acidic group at one end.

The first of the omega-3 fatty acids is alpha linolenic acid, or ALA, the single parent of this family of fats. Found primarily in the leaves and other green parts of plants, alpha linolenic acid is the fat associated with the complex photosynthetic machinery of plants, the fat that enables plants to capture single photons of light and turn them into sugars, the basis of all life on earth. Alpha linolenic acid doesn't play a significant role in animals, for reasons I will soon discuss, but it does give rise to offspring who do work that is every bit as important to animals as photosynthesis is to plants.

Like all fatty acids, alpha linolenic acid is a weak acid—that is, it has a slight tendency to lose a hydrogen ion and develop a negative charge. It has the same strength as a very familiar acid, vinegar, which is not surprising since vinegar, or acetic acid, is also a fatty acid that is common in living tissues but too short (just two carbons long) to be of use in storing energy or building structures.

Fatty acids lose their acidic leaning when they team up with a molecule of glycerol to make triglycerides, the substances we commonly call fats (the substances we cook with and that don't mix with water). In most contexts, we can think of *fatty acids* and *fats* as equivalent terms. And we can think of the acidic end of a fatty acid as the hook, or the coupling, that enables our bodies to move these long, sticky chains of carbons and hydrogens around.

It's helpful to understand that all triglycerides have an identical glycerol backbone attached to three, often different, fatty acids, sixteen to twenty-two carbons in length.

1 glycerol + 3 fatty acids → 1 triglyceride + 3 molecules water

Whether these triglycerides take the shape of butter, vegetable oil, lard, or suet depends entirely on which fatty acids are involved. Some fatty acids have straight, saturated chains (saturated with hydrogens, that is) and produce solid fats; others have kinky, unsaturated chains (where some of the hydrogens have been replaced by double bonds between the carbons) and produce liquids.

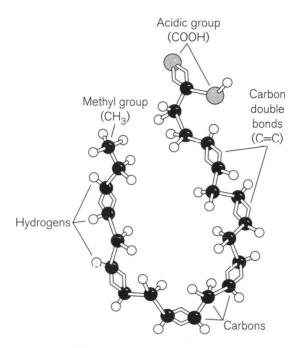

Acidic group
(COOH)

Methyl group
(CH₃)

Carbon
double
bonds
(C=C)

Hydrogens

Carbons

FIGURE 1 DHA in one of its many conformations. Sometimes this fatty acid curls up in a ball; sometimes it is as straight as a ruler. Its six double bonds keep it constantly on the move.

Alpha linolenic acid has a markedly kinky tail, and the fats in which it is abundant—linseed, canola, and soybean oils—are liquids, even at very low temperatures. But alpha linolenic acid is not kinky enough for animals, which are faster (more mobile) than plants, and animals lengthen and add double bonds to this eighteen-carbon fatty acid before they put it to work in their tissues.

Docosahexaenoic acid, or DHA, is one of several offspring of alpha linolenic acid and it is the longest, most desaturated fatty acid in animal tissues. It is the fat that permits animals to think and see. DHA is found in its highest concentrations in the membranes of the cells of the brain and eyes, where its ability to flip-flop between hundreds of different shapes, billions of times per second—the result of an extremely kinky chain with six carbon double bonds (twice as many as in alpha linolenic acid)—enables nerve cells to send their rapid signals. DHA is a quick-change artist, scientists have recently learned, and its concentrated presence in cell membranes, the thin envelopes surrounding cells, transforms those barriers from orderly guards into dancers at an all-night rave. Its dilute presence in cells throughout the body is like oil added to an engine.

Animals make very different use of a second, somewhat shorter, offspring of alpha linolenic acid: eicosapentaenoic acid. Eicosapentaenoic acid, or EPA, is one of several fatty acids, all twenty carbons long, that animal cells release from their membranes in order to communicate with each other and affect each other's behavior (fat signals instead of smoke signals). I'll talk more about these cell messengers later—how they were discovered and what kinds of reactions they produce—but the reader should know that this kind of communication is necessary in any organism with more than one cell and that eicosapentaenoic stands out as the mediator or peacemaker of these fat messengers. When this omega-3 fatty acid is released from a cell, it produces just the kind of measured reaction in its neighbors that is desirable in most family or neighborly interactions. It does not elicit the extreme reactions of other fat messengers—say, arachidonic acid, which enters the scene like a SWAT team. Sending in a SWAT team can be useful in some situations (in fighting infection, for example), but not to coordinate everyday disagreements.

The omega-3 fats are not rare in nature, as their remarkable behaviors might lead us to think. In fact, alpha linolenic acid, found in the chloroplasts of green leaves, is the most abundant fat on earth. Green leaves are not known for being fatty, high-calorie foods; but the planet has more green vegetation on it than anything else, and the small amount of fat in each leaf adds up. DHA and eicosapentaenoic acid* are also common, since these offspring of alpha linolenic acid accumulate in the tissues of animals that eat green leaves, as well as in the tissues of animals that eat the animals that eat green leaves. Both DHA and eicosapentaenoic acid are also made by some aquatic plants.

But these fats have become rare in most Americans' diets, which are short on leafy greens and long on seeds and the oil

*To those wondering about my inconsistency in referring to these fatty acids, using the acronym for docosahexaenoic acid, DHA, but writing out alpha linolenic acid and eicosapentaenoic acid—it is intentional. I didn't want the reader thinking of the American Library Association (ALA) or the Environmental Protection Agency (EPA) every time I used their accepted acronyms. But DHA, as far as I know, doesn't stand for any familiar organization, and the use of at least one acronym may be helpful in keeping these fats straight. When I introduce the members of the omega-6 family of fats, I will be more consistent and spell each of them out. The abbreviation for arachidonic acid used by the scientific community is AA, and I don't want anyone's mind going to Alcoholics Anonymous. Or to Los Angeles, since LA is the abbreviation of linoleic acid, the parent of this second family. I will be inconsistent throughout the book, however, in using a combination of common and scientific names for these fatty acids, whichever seems to be the most reader-friendly. The common names reflect the discovery of these compounds—oleic acid was first isolated from olive oil; linolenic acid, from linseed oil—and are sometimes less cumbersome than their scientific equivalents (here, octadecenoic and octadecatrienoic acid, respectively). But the names derived from Greek or Latin—eicosapentaenoic acid, for example—have the advantage of giving the number of carbons and double bonds and are sometimes easier to remember.

from seeds, including soybeans and corn. And this rarity—this deficiency or insufficiency, as people have been calling it since the 1980s—is now being linked to a whole host of human ills. These include diseases of the brain, because of the high concentration of DHA in healthy nervous tissue, as well as heart disease, arthritis and other inflammatory diseases, certain kinds of cancers, and metabolic diseases such as obesity and diabetes, the diseases that tend to specifically plague Western populations—the diseases of civilization, as they have been called, without irony.

Scientists do not know everything there is to know about this family of fats and how their absence from the human diet causes disease—far from it. But what they do know should make physicians and government agencies sit up and take notice before uttering another word of dietary advice. It should cause a thorough reevaluation of our guidelines about fats and health. Why it hasn't is a good question and has something to do with resistance on the part of food industries (which have been removing omega-3s from foods because the many double bonds in omega-3 fats make them more easily oxidized than other fats, resulting in a shorter shelf life for the products that contain them), as well as with the complexity of the science that is involved. (Who would have ever thought that something as lumpish as fat could be so complicated?) It may also have something to do with the slow, meandering history of our understanding of these fats and with our very gradual realization that a balance of the different fats is essential for health.

Which brings me to the reason I have written this book: that the telling of this history may help us to see how omega-3s came to be eliminated from both our diets and our nutritional thinking and to discover how to put them back. A recounting of the ideas that shaped research and dominated medicine may reveal where the advice given us went wrong and give us the courage to make amends. This book is a tribute to the missing fats in our diet. It is also the history of how researchers discovered that these fats were missing—a nutritional whodunit that plays out in Greenland, Africa, and the many Western countries whose inhabitants first experienced this absence in the form of an epidemic of heart disease.

For many reasons, we have arrived at a critical time for this history. Though for decades we have been advised to consume diets that are low in cholesterol and saturated fat (avoiding foods such as butter and lard, which have a high percentage of straight, saturated chains), and though cholesterol and saturated fat have been reduced in the American diet, heart disease continues to afflict just as many Americans—and we're now facing epidemics of obesity and diabetes. Saturated fat and cholesterol were supposed to be the problem, so where did we go wrong? Why are our health woes multiplying instead of going away? Many explanations for this unhealthy trend have been proposed, including larger portion sizes, excess calories, an increase in the consumption of processed carbohydrates and trans fats, and a decrease in exercise, all of which may share some of the responsibility. But it's time we learned that certain fats—the fats in most of our foods—slow down metabolism, as researchers in Australia are finding. It's time we learned that many companies, in processing food, routinely eliminate the omega-3 fats that are important to both maintaining energy balance and protecting the heart.

A new labeling policy instituted in the United States, effective January 1, 2006, requires food producers to state the amount of trans fats in their products. Such labels are a good thing, since they will enable consumers to avoid these altered fats, which result from a hydrogenation process that makes vegetable oils more solid and stable (that is, less susceptible to oxidation). But the labels won't do much if food producers substitute fats that are just as unhealthy as trans fats, which is how the food industry seems to be handling the trans hysteria.

Recognizing that the public usually focuses on one bad guy at a time, food manufacturers have replaced trans fats with saturated or monounsaturated fats, or with polyunsaturated fats of the omega-6 family. These polyunsaturates also have multiple double bonds (though somewhat fewer than omega-3s, thereby making them more stable) and are also essential for health, but they compete with omega-3s for places in our cells and membranes and have very different effects on human health, as research has clearly shown. It is time we stopped thinking about good guys and bad guys, good fats and bad fats, and developed a more nuanced outlook toward these underappreciated and frequently maligned nutrients, understanding that all fats play a role in human nutrition and that disease is caused by imbalances between them, not by their mere presence in our diet.

At the same time, biologists are now able to genetically modify plants to produce many different kinds of fats. They are close to being able to insert into spinach the genes used by marine plants in making DHA, for example. Some of these engineered plants will be a boon to health, since they will be able to restore fats that are missing in the diet. Others will be new to human bodies, or available in amounts never seen before, and their effect on the body (over time) is anyone's guess. Scientists are also altering the cooking and salad oils that are familiar to us, using conventional hybridizing techniques as well as genetic modification, and some of the new oils do not live up to their old reputations.

Take canola oil, for instance, an oil that is associated with good health because it is high in alpha linolenic acid, the parent omega-3. Canola oil, which was introduced into the United States in 1985, has been single-handedly responsible for a small increase in the omega-3 content of our diet in recent decades.

Meanwhile plant biologists have been developing low alpha linolenic strains of rapeseed, the plant whose seeds are used to produce canola oil, just as they have developed low alpha linolenic strains of soybeans. The new strains produce oils that are less susceptible to oxidation and might not require hydrogenation, but they are also less beneficial.

Another pressing reason for this history is the confusion and concern about contamination of fish with mercury and PCBs (polychlorinated biphenyls). Pregnant and nursing women are in a terrible quandary. They are told that the fats in fish will help their infant's brain, eyes, and heart to develop properly; yet mercury is known to cause neurological damage. They are advised to consume two meals of fish a week but warned that they should avoid albacore tuna or eat no more than 6 ounces of it a week, advice that is off-putting to even the biggest fans of fish. The issue of PCBs is just as perplexing, with the Food and Drug Administration saying that they pose no threat to most fish supplies and environmental groups urging caution.

Those who are neither pregnant nor nursing worry about contaminants as well, and any thinking person must be concerned about the health of our seas and the sustainability of our fish resources (especially if the advice to eat fish twice a week is taken seriously). At a time when more than 70 percent of commercial fish stocks are said to be "fully exploited, overfished or collapsed," it's critical for us to understand that eating fish is not the only way to increase our intake of omega-3s. Nor is it the most effective way, as I will explain. Protecting our seas and waters is important for many reasons, but simply eating fish cannot solve this nutritional problem.

This history is also timely because many of the researchers who first reported the problem associated with omega-3s are retired from their laboratories, or close to retiring. But they were still very much alive and able to tell me their stories when I visited them in Minnesota, Copenhagen, London, and Washington and when they spoke to me by phone from Ohio, Sweden, Italy, and Canada. They know firsthand how different fats behave in the cells of our bodies. They collected data showing that people in America and other Western countries have greatly reduced the amounts of omega-3s in their bodies, and they began linking those reductions to illnesses like heart disease. Others have expanded on that work to reveal how omega-3s operate in healthy, well-nourished people and to describe the special role of DHA in dynamic, fast-acting cells like neurons and heart muscle.

I end this introduction, then, with a few more examples of where DHA is found in humans and other animals, examples that speak to the new and growing understanding that DHA, the longest and most unsaturated omega-3, is required for life's speediest tasks.

In human bodies, as I've already noted, the tissues with the most DHA are the tissues of the brain and the eyes, including the eyes that are focused on this page. The second-highest concentration of DHA is found in sperm, which have to swim the fastest, most competitive race of all; next is heart muscle, which beats seventy times per minute, some two billion times in a lifetime.

DHA is found in lesser amounts throughout the rest of the human body, and there its concentrations are influenced by exercise and genetics, as well as diet. Athletes trained for endurance have much more DHA in their skeletal muscle than do less-active individuals. The Pima Indians of Arizona, a population with the highest reported incidence of type 2, or non-insulin-dependent, diabetes, have much *less* DHA in their skeletal muscle than other populations, a finding that scientists attribute to genetic differences.

In hummingbirds, some of life's speediest creatures, the flight muscles, which beat *fifty-two times per second*, are extremely rich in DHA; the leg muscles are not.* In rattlesnakes, the high-frequency rattle muscle has much more DHA than the low-frequency stomach muscle.

Reptiles, in general, have lower levels of DHA in their tissues than do mammals and birds (and lower metabolic rates); and fish have higher levels, which is understandable since fish live under pressure, in cold, dim environments. They need greater flexibility in their membranes, *and* they have ready access to algae and other high omega-3 foods.

Finally, caribou, which walk the frozen tundra of the far north, have more DHA in their hooves than in their upper legs, which improves the circulation of those parts in direct contact with the permafrost. And hibernating animals, like the yellow-bellied marmot from Colorado, have much *less* DHA in their tissues when they are hibernating than when they are awake. It's not that they lose DHA as they sleep; rather, their bodies do not slow down and go into hibernation when their diet is rich in omega-3s.

*Hummingbirds eat more than nectar, in case the reader is wondering where they get all this DHA. With their beaks agape, they nab insects (a source of DHA) in the air.

TWO

A TRIP TO GREENLAND

Oh, call it not blubber!

DR. ELISHA KENT KANE, POLAR EXPLORER

DHA, THE QUICK-CHANGE ARTIST, WAS NOT THE FIRST OMEGA-3 FATTY acid to catch the attention of scientists. Their interest and concern had earlier been aroused by eicosapentaenoic acid, the fat I called the mediator or peacemaker of cell messengers. Eicosapentaenoic acid, whose name describes the makeup of its molecule—twenty (*eikosi*, in Greek) carbons and five *(penta)* double bonds—was made a celebrity in the 1970s after two Danish physicians got it into their heads to go to Greenland and investigate stories they had heard about the Eskimos' lack of heart disease. This absence was curious, these doctors thought, because the Eskimos, also known as the Inuit, eat a lot of blubber and fat. And isn't fat the dietary demon that causes this disease?

Heart disease, or angina pectoris, the condition that laypeople sometimes call hardening of the arteries, because it is often marked by the lining of the arteries filling with the waxy substance cholesterol, and physicians sometimes call *morbus medicorum* (illness of doctors), because it so frequently strikes those in the medical profession, was almost unknown at the beginning of the twentieth century. But by the middle of the century it was the number one killer in countries such as Denmark and the United States—a status it would maintain, at least in America, until 2004, when it was bested by deaths from cancer. The heart attack that President Dwight D. Eisenhower suffered in 1955 while on vacation in Denver galvanized Americans to seek out the reasons for this strange and sudden upswing.

In the 1960s, one large epidemiological study (the Framingham Study) established a link between the amount of cholesterol in a person's blood and his or her risk for heart disease; another (the Seven Countries Study) connected a population's incidence of heart disease and its cholesterol levels to the percentage of calories consumed as fat.

These associations were far from perfect, though. Some populations, including the Greeks, consumed large amounts of fat and had a low incidence of heart disease; and some individuals had low serum cholesterol levels yet died of heart attacks. As new ways of screening blood for fats in addition to cholesterol were being invented and refined, many physicians hoped that these new tests—such as those for triglycerides (the form in which plants and animals store fats), phospholipids (the building blocks of cell membranes), and lipoproteins (the protein-lipid complexes that transport fats within animals)—would be of even greater predictive value.

Among them were two Danish physicians who intended to start a clinic in the northern city of Ålborg to treat patients with hyperlipidemia, or excessive amounts of fats in their blood. Hans Olaf Bang, a colorful figure known as "H.O." who smoked a pipe and wore a beret and long gray cape, and Jørn Dyerberg, one of his young residents, had all the newest methods for screening blood and were prepared to use them.

But in May 1969 Bang read something that changed the course, and the place, of their research. In an editorial published in the *Ugeskrift for Læger*, a weekly publication for physicians that is the Danish equivalent of the *Journal of the American Medical Association (JAMA)* and the oldest medical journal in the world, a doctor who had spent a lot of time in Greenland, a self-governing province of Denmark, remarked on the fact that Eskimos died from tuberculosis and infection—but not diseases of the arteries. The piece caught Bang's attention because of his current interests, of course, but also because he had been looking for a way to return to Greenland since the 1950s, when as a young doctor he had treated a measles epidemic there. "He had lost his heart to Greenland," Dyerberg now recalls of his colleague, who died in 1994, "like so many who visit that place."

So when Bang read the editorial, he turned to Dyerberg and said, "Let's go. Let's go to Greenland and see how their blood lipids are." He was intrigued by the apparent contradiction in the Eskimos, who were known for consuming large amounts of seal and whale blubber, and he didn't know, or didn't care, that Ancel Keys, one of the preeminent researchers in the field and the head investigator of the Seven Countries Study, had already dismissed their experience as in any way weakening the link between fat consumption and heart disease. "The fish industry is heartened by imaginative statements that coronary heart-disease is absent in Eskimos and rare in Norwegians because of their consumption of marine oils," Keys wrote with characteristic certitude in a 1957 paper published in the British medical journal *Lancet*, "though actually the incidence of coronary heart-disease among Eskimos is entirely unknown and the disease is anything but rare in Norway."

Bang instantly decided to follow up on the editorial, and he and Dyerberg began planning for the trip. Because they were not well-known researchers, raising the money they required was no easy matter. They started by collecting all the medical records they could find from Greenland—some 2,000 of them; from these, they calculated that the death rate from heart disease was indeed much lower in Greenland than in Denmark—no more than a tenth as great. They then used that information to persuade the Danish Heart Association, as well as a bank in the city of Ålborg and private donors, to fund them; in all, they collected $10,000.

During this time, Bang and Dyerberg had already begun seeking advice from physicians in Greenland about the best place for their study. They wanted access to Eskimos who still lived by hunting and fishing, since they suspected that the Eskimos' protection from heart disease had something to do with the unusually high concentration of fish and meat in their diet. But the doctors required access to a laboratory where they could analyze their blood samples. Lipoproteins, the complexes that move fat around the body, break down within twenty-four hours, as they knew, so they had to run those tests immediately.

(Why fats require this kind of chaperoning may not be immediately obvious to readers, so I'll interrupt the story to briefly explain. It is because unaccompanied fats are insoluble in the watery soup of our blood and would stick to the walls of cells and vessels. The body must disguise fats in order to move them around—wolves in sheep's clothing—by tucking them inside proteins that are hydrophobic on the inside but water soluble on the outside. This sounds and is complicated: these complexes must be disassembled and reassembled every time fats cross from one cell or tissue into another, a process that involves numerous receptors and proteins. But the payoff is the extra energy provided by fats—9 calories per gram, as compared to about 4 for carbohydrates and proteins—and a watertight building material that can be used to form the membranes of cells.)

Eventually, Bang and Dyerberg decided on the small town of Umanak, on Greenland's west coast, because it had seven small

Eskimo settlements within a distance of just 100 kilometers and its twenty-bed hospital—the northernmost hospital in Greenland—had a tiny lab with electricity. They didn't know it at the time, but Umanak, which is on an inlet of Baffin Bay, means "heart" in Inuktitut; it was named for the unusual heart-shaped mountain outside town. "It can't get better than that," says Dyerberg today.

On the first of what would turn out to be five trips to Greenland, Bang, Dyerberg, and Aase Brøndum Nielsen, their technician, planned to simply measure the blood fats in a group of traditional Greenlanders, whom they would then compare to a group of Danes living in Greenland (but consuming a typical Danish diet of dairy products and pork) and to Eskimos living in Denmark. They would go in late August, the best time for traveling by sailboat in the fjords of the west coast of Greenland and a time of year when hunting and fishing are good, ensuring that the Eskimos would be eating their traditional diet of halibut, seal, and whale meat, including large amounts of seal and whale blubber.

Indeed, that diet was at the center of the puzzle that Bang and Dyerberg hoped to unravel. Since the Eskimos' consumption of fat was high, would their blood lipids also be high? If the answer was yes, then the power of blood lipid levels to predict heart disease would be put in question; if no, then widely accepted recommendations to reduce intake of fat, especially animal fat, would be undercut.

The three Danes flew from Denmark to the American base at Søndre Strømfjord on Greenland's west coast, then traveled north on a boat carrying passengers, whale meat, and other cargo. In the waters outside Umanak, a porter from the hospital met them and transferred them and their belongings to a much smaller sailboat—the same boat that would later take them to the Eskimo settlements.

Thus began a wonderful three weeks, Dyerberg and Nielsen agree, as they sailed to one after another of the outlying communities. There, they spent time drinking coffee and talking (with the help of a translator) to the residents, persuading at least some of them to allow their blood to be drawn in the morning, before the Eskimos ate and before the three researchers had to sail back to Umanak to run their tests. On the nights the researchers were away from Umanak, they slept wherever they could: in a corner of a store, in a school, or in a church. In Umanak, the three of them shared a room in the hospital.

"We were like scouts," Nielsen said when I called her at her home in Denmark, "and besides, the long arctic days weren't much for sleeping." Instead of sleeping, they laughed a lot, played poker, walked on the beach at 2:00 A.M., and talked about their work. Bang sketched the ever-changing panorama of icebergs, as well as the Eskimos' tools and houses. Soon, Dyerberg and Nielsen were losing their hearts to Greenland, as Bang already had. "There was absolutely no sound when you moved away from the towns," remembers Nielsen. "No sound and then you have the sky which goes up, up and never ends and the sea which goes down, down and never ends. You feel like a little dot in the universe."

The only thing Nielsen didn't like was seal meat, which was the usual fare. Dyerberg liked seal meat, when it was fried, but was unnerved by the hundreds of sled dogs that ran free and foraged for themselves during the summer. In one of the communities they visited, there were 95 people and about 950 dogs. Dyerberg always carried a large stone for self-defense.

The people themselves were curious and friendly, though shockingly poor in Nielsen's eyes, and with terrible teeth from their habit of sipping their coffee through a sugar cube. "They had so little," Nielsen recalls, "just their clothes, tools, dogs, and a small house built of stones and turf. But they had very good senses of humor and were very helpful to us." One hundred thirty Eskimos, sixty-one men and sixty-nine women, wound up volunteering for the study. Nielsen was the first to suspect that something was very different about the blood that coursed through their veins. She was in charge of drawing it in the morning, and she noticed right away how long it took for the Eskimos to stop bleeding: not two to four minutes, as was the case for most Danes (and most Americans), but at least twice that long. Nielsen was not then aware of the Eskimos' reputation for having frequent nosebleeds, and only later would Bang and Dyerberg begin to wonder whether the Eskimos' "bleeding time," as it is called, and their low incidence of heart disease were connected.

Immediately after collecting the blood, Nielsen drew off the plasma. Then, within twelve hours, she or her colleagues placed samples of the plasma onto gel strips and ran them through their electrophoresis machine. This separated the lipoproteins into three classes according to their density. These were the low-density lipoproteins, or LDLs (beta lipoproteins, as they were then known); the very-low-density lipoproteins, or VLDLs (pre-beta lipoproteins); and the high-density lipoproteins, or HDLs (alpha lipoproteins). The rest of the volunteers' plasma was frozen and brought back to Denmark, where tests that did not need to be performed immediately—analysis for total lipid content, cholesterol, phospholipids, and triglycerides—were carried out.

These were all the tests that were routinely carried out at that time, and they showed that levels of all the lipoproteins, except HDL, were clearly and significantly lower in the Greenland Eskimos than in the Danes. The same was true of all the lipids (except the phospholipids, whose levels were the same). This outcome was not surprising, given the Eskimos' low incidence of heart disease, but it was surprising in light of their diet rich in animal fat and cholesterol. Moreover, it seemed to be the result of dietary rather than genetic differences, since Eskimos living in Denmark had lipid profiles resembling those of Danes.

In their paper in the *Lancet*, Bang, Dyerberg, and Nielsen suggested that the explanation was "probably the large amount of polyunsaturated fatty acids in the fat tissue of the animals eaten," since polyunsaturated fats were known, by that time, to protect against increases in levels of plasma cholesterol. They were just guessing that the fat tissue of whales and seals was high in polyunsaturates; unlike today, at the time nothing was known about the fats of most fish and marine mammals. But they based their guess both on the information available regarding the fats in a fish that had been analyzed, salmon, and on a belief that "the composition of animal fatty tissue changes more and more in the polyunsaturated direction as the temperature of the medium in which the animal lives decreases."

That same paper, which Dyerberg says was a "mere curiosity" when first published but has since been labeled by *Nutrition Reviews* a "nutrition classic," was the very first to record the presence of a high concentration of high-density lipoproteins in a population with a low incidence of heart disease. HDLs are what many today know as "good cholesterol" because they remove excess and damaged lipids (mostly cholesterol) from cells, bringing them back to the liver for reuse or excretion. They are dense because they are mostly protein. Relative to LDLs and VLDLs, the lipoproteins that collect fats after a meal and deliver them to tissues, they carry small lipid loads and are therefore more soluble in blood.

The Danish researchers' next step—their "next stroke of luck," as Dyerberg calls it—was to analyze the 130 frozen samples they had brought back with them from Greenland in even greater depth. They decided to look at the basic building blocks of the lipids in the Eskimos' blood—the fifty or so different fatty acids, both saturated and unsaturated, that the body uses to construct its triglycerides and phospholipids and to esterify (or link) to cholesterol. Most of the cholesterol in the body, including the cholesterol in the plaque that forms on artery walls, is linked to one or another fatty acid.

Bang and Dyerberg had the type of machine needed for such analysis, a gas-liquid chromatograph that they had acquired for their new clinic but had hardly ever used. Gas-liquid chromatography had been developed in the 1950s by oil companies to provide a kind of chemical fingerprint when they suspected that people were diluting their high-quality oil with cheaper stuff, but it had been quickly adopted by the biomedical community to use in analyzing fats. Not until the invention of gas-liquid chromatography could all the individual fatty acids that make up fats and oils be separated and measured, making it possible for researchers to begin to appreciate the qualities and effects of each. In this device, fatty acids are separated on the basis of their boiling point, a function of their molecular weight as well as of the number and type of double bonds. Short, saturated fatty acids come through the long column of the chromatograph first. Longer ones come later, and long, unsaturated fatty acids come in last. As a particular compound passes through the column, it is burned over a flame, generating a signal that is recorded as a peak or spike.

"I guess no one else is going to be collecting samples from Eskimos living from hunting and fishing anytime soon," Dyerberg remembers Bang saying. "So let's do whatever we can with these samples and publish the data so it is out there for anyone to see. The world is changing, so let's let people know that in 1970, the Eskimos looked like this." Those words were prophetic, since the difference in the incidence of heart disease in Greenland and in Western countries such as Denmark and the United States would disappear almost completely within two decades, after the Eskimos adopted many aspects of a Western diet.

The decision to "do whatever we can" with the samples was also wise, since the results of these in-depth studies were immediately intriguing. When Dyerberg and Bang separated out and measured all the different fatty acids in the lipids of Eskimos and Danes, they found striking differences in the two populations. In particular, the Eskimos' blood contained very small amounts of an unsaturated fatty acid that Dyerberg and Bang identified as arachidonic acid (so named in 1913 because it is the same length as arachidic acid, a saturated fat found in peanuts, but has multiple double bonds) and very large amounts of a fatty acid that they could not identify. This unidentifiable fatty acid showed up near the very end of the graph, indicating that it was either longer than arachidonic acid or more unsaturated. The Eskimos had seven times as much of this mystery fat as did Danes, and about one-seventh the amount of arachidonic acid.

Dyerberg and Bang knew that arachidonic acid was an elongated offspring of linoleic acid, the only fat known at the time to be essential for human health. In order to find out what the mystery fat was, they decided that Dyerberg should fly to the United States and visit Ralph Holman, a world authority on fats who worked at the Hormel Institute in Austin, Minnesota, about 80 miles south of St. Paul.

Holman had been one of the first to use the powerful new technique of gas-liquid chromatography to study the fats in animal tissues, and he was able to quickly identify the large spike on Dyerberg's graph as eicosapentaenoic acid, a fatty acid that has the same number of carbons as arachidonic acid (twenty) but one more double bond. He also identified a second, smaller spike at the tail end of the graph as DHA. This spike was also larger in Eskimos than in Danes, though the spike was much smaller and the difference was not as great.

So it was the large amount of eicosapentaenoic acid in the blood of Eskimos that caught Dyerberg's attention—and imagination. As he left Holman's lab, he remembers saying the word over and over again. "Ei-co . . . Ei-co-sa . . . eicosapentaenoic acid."

THREE

HOW THE OMEGAS GOT THEIR NAME

I am Alpha and Omega, the beginning and the end.

REVELATION 1:8, 21:6

WHAT JØRN DYERBERG AND RALPH HOLMAN DID NOT DISCUSS, AS far as either of them can remember, was Holman's work over the past three decades, work that revealed the competition between fatty acids such as arachidonic acid and eicosapentaenoic acid for enzymes and for coveted spots in the membranes of cells. This discussion would have put Dyerberg and Bang's unusual findings about Eskimos into a broader context and might even have led to an earlier understanding of the role of omega-3s in healthy diets.

Holman showed Dyerberg around the Hormel Institute where he worked (it is somewhat ironic that the most important work on unsaturated fatty acids was funded by the company that makes the highly saturated meat product Spam). But for some reason, perhaps because Dyerberg was already overloaded with new information, they did not talk about this competition, or about how Holman and his graduate students had deduced this metabolic rivalry, painstakingly and brilliantly, from feeding experiments in rats.

Eating fish helps prevent heart disease. That was the medical advice that emerged out of Dyerberg and Bang's trips to Greenland. But the effectiveness of fish depends very much, as an understanding of Holman's work would have made clear, on what other fats are hanging around the body. Will the fats in fish have a chance to become the building materials and messengers of cells? Or will they be swamped, outnumbered and overwhelmed by different kinds of fats?

Dyerberg left Holman's lab with standards for both eicosapentaenoic acid and DHA, two fats that are more abundant in the blood of heart-healthy Eskimos than in that of Danes. But he didn't go home with an appreciation that "the metabolism of unsaturated acids is influenced by the concentrations and kinds of other fatty acids present in the diet and in the metabolic pool," as Holman wrote in 1964. Or that "the concept of balanced diet must include a consideration of balanced concentrations of the several polyunsaturated, monounsaturated and saturated fatty acids."

His lack of appreciation isn't altogether surprising, since most physicians have yet to grasp this important concept. The nutritional guidelines of the United States Department of Agriculture don't mention it in their most recent dietary recommendations. Instead, one after another of the fats in the food supply has been vilified (saturated and animal fats in the 1960s, tropical oils in the 1980s, trans fats in the 1990s), until the public has become so confused, disbelieving, and rebellious that it now indulges in all fats. We could have spared ourselves a lot of trouble and heartache (as well as other heart problems) if we had incorporated Holman's findings earlier on. But to do so might have required that we learn some fairly complicated things about fats. And it is probably true, as Alexis de Tocqueville once remarked, that Americans prefer a simple lie to a complex truth.

Ralph Holman, the son of a streetcar driver in Minneapolis and the grandson, on both sides, of Swedish immigrants to Upsala,

Minnesota, has spent most of his life thinking about fats. His interest in the subject began in 1943, when his first thesis project, a study of sugar metabolism, was derailed by the Second World War and the beginnings of the Manhattan Project. This covert operation corralled many of the scientists who were experienced in working with radioactive materials, including a member of the University of Minnesota's Department of Physics. Suddenly—in fact, overnight—Holman was left without a source of radioactive glucose, a key ingredient of his studies. Exempted from war duty himself because he was teaching physicians and nurses at the University of Minnesota and because he was underweight for his height (when he tried to enlist, he was told to come back after gaining 40 pounds), Holman went to his thesis advisor, George Burr, for a new project; and Burr suggested that he try his hand at fats.

Fats had always been a research interest of Burr's, the one for which he is best remembered, but he had been forced to put them on the back burner for want of the right techniques with which to isolate and study them.

More than a decade earlier, in 1929, Burr and his wife, Mildred, made nutritional history by showing that fat is an essential nutrient for rats. Without fat in their diet, the Burrs had found, rats develop a scaly skin and lose considerable amounts of weight—even though their caloric intake is more than sufficient for health. After a period of months, their tails begin to swell and die back, and their kidneys degenerate, allowing the passage of blood in their urine. Neither males nor females are able to reproduce. Unless these fat-deprived rats are given certain fats—the fat in lard, for instance, but not the fat in coconut oil—they will die at an early age. If they are given a small amount of the right fat, "the cure is as spectacular as those cures produced by the well known vitamins," the Burrs wrote.

It's hard to imagine that this finding was ever very controversial, but in 1929 the belief that fats perform no other function than that of providing energy or delivering fat-soluble vitamins was thoroughly entrenched in scientific doctrine. Because fat can be made from carbohydrates, a reaction known since the middle of the nineteenth century, scientists and nutritionists thought that fat can't be essential in the way that vitamins and amino acids are essential. What they were overlooking is that the fats the body is able to make from scratch are harder and less fluid, more saturated with hydrogen atoms, than some of the fats found in nature—the fat of pigs or fish, for example. This belief in the nonessentialness of fat was so strong, even in Burr and his wife, that it took this scientific couple four years to correctly interpret their experiments.

Once they did, and the term *essential fatty acid* was born, follow-up experiments were hampered by the lack of any good methods for purifying unsaturated fatty acids and measuring the amounts of different fatty acids in tissues. The Burrs were certain that linoleic acid, a fatty acid with two double bonds that is found (in increasing amounts) in olive oil, lard, corn oil, and poppy seed oil, was an essential fat since it could completely cure the problems of rats on a fat-free diet. (A helpful way to remember the difference between linoleic acid and the very similar-sounding linolenic acid is that the word *linoleic* has one fewer letter—and the acid has one fewer double bond.) But they were confused about the essentialness of arachidonic acid. They didn't know at the time that arachidonic acid is made from linoleic acid (by a two-carbon elongation and the insertion of two double bonds). So why, they wondered, should it have such a potent effect when it was not found in any of the oils that contained linoleic acid?

Fatty acids with three double bonds, or linolenic acids, were also baffling to the Burrs, and their confusion about the essentialness of these fats—the most prevalent form of which is alpha linolenic acid, the parent omega-3 fat—has had a long-lasting effect on the field. The reason the Burrs thought linolenic acid might be essential was that linseed oil (which is rich in alpha linolenic acid) was able to remedy the deficiency in their rats. But linseed oil is also rich in linoleic acid and that, as scientists who later were able to separate these fats finally understood, was the active component in the Burrs' experiments. Rats do require alpha linolenic acid, as others showed still later, but it is much more difficult to make a rat deficient in this and other omega-3 fats, since rats (and other animals) cling to these fats tenaciously. It can be done, but it takes much longer than it does to produce a linoleic acid deficiency.

The results of those follow-up experiments that the Burrs could undertake in the 1930s were also confusing and took decades to comprehend fully. Their attempt to prove that linoleic acid was essential for humans as well as rats by putting a friend of theirs on a fat-free diet for six months failed, we now know, because the fat reserves of an average human contain approximately 2 pounds of linoleic acid. Those 2 pounds take much longer than six months to deplete. Adult rats begin showing signs of linoleic acid deficiency only after several months; healthy adult humans take much longer.

The Burrs' volunteer for this experiment, a biochemist named William Redman Brown, was clinically well throughout the experiment, though his meals were restricted to sucrose, potato starch, special skim milk, orange juice, salts, vitamins, and flavoring matter. He never even had a cold, and scientists concluded—incorrectly—that linoleic acid was essential for rats, but it was not essential for humans. Essentiality in humans was finally proven in the 1960s when intravenous feeding, or total parenteral nutrition (TPN), was developed as a way of maintaining patients during surgery and hospitalization. The first TPN preparations were fat-free, and patients on them for long periods developed symptoms (scaly skin, etc.) that looked a lot like those of the Burrs' rats. By then, the Burrs had moved to Hawaii to study pineapple cultivation and had left the field entirely.

George Burr, in other words, had many good reasons for putting the question of essential fatty acids on the back burner of his scientific stove in the 1930s and focusing instead on how sugar is metabolized. But in 1943, when Ralph Holman approached him for a new project, he had recently acquired an instrument, an advanced spectrophotometer, and saw an opportunity for using it to probe more deeply into fats. Fatty acids with different numbers and arrangements of double bonds would absorb different amounts of ultraviolet light, he thought, and might allow some of the unanswered questions to be addressed. Plus, Burr probably saw in Holman, an unassuming man who had built most of the furniture in his house, the kind of resourcefulness that would enable him to invent whatever techniques and build whatever equipment he needed to move forward.

Thus Holman became a grease monkey, a fat guy, a guru of grease, as he joked at eighty-three (he is, in fact, still very lean). The Hormel Company, which had been funding George Burr since 1938, had an interest in fat oxidation, which goes up exponentially with the number of double bonds in fats and is the major cause of rancidity in foods. So Burr gave Holman the task of studying this topic. And Holman turned this modest assignment into a life's career with a tremendous impact on human health. He is grateful "to have been set loose in a field where there was little knowledge and little competition—and the opportunities were therefore the greatest."

When Holman entered the fat arena, the only fat in which anyone was interested, as far as human health was concerned, was cholesterol. Essential fats had been found (incorrectly) to be required only by rats, and cholesterol, first isolated from gallstones in the early 1800s, grabbed all the attention because it was the first fat that could be measured. Found exclusively in animal tissues, cholesterol turns a convenient blue-green color when it is treated with a strong acid (specifically, a mixture of sulfuric and acetic acids). When Holman entered graduate school in chemistry in 1941, his laboratory manual contained only one procedure related to fats: the Liebermann-Burchard method for determining cholesterol.

Holman wasn't interested in cholesterol, though, because humans, and other animals, could make it themselves. They consumed it every time they ate meat and fat, but their livers could also manufacture it out of any two-carbon fragment that came their way. It wasn't like those polyunsaturated fats that the body couldn't make, fats that had to be consumed via plants (or via animals that eat plants). Two scientists using heavy hydrogen as a biological tag had conclusively demonstrated this inability. "In contrast to all other fatty acids investigated so far, linoleic and linolenic do not take up deuterium from the heavy water of body fluids," Rudolf Schoenheimer and David Rittenberg reported in 1940. "These highly unsaturated acids must have been derived from the diet."

Holman's first task, the same task that had stumped Burr a decade earlier, was to prepare pure samples of all the individual polyunsaturated fatty acids. This meant isolating one fatty acid—alpha linolenic acid, for example—from the messy soup of fatty acids that constitutes every fat or oil, however homogeneous and uniform these substances may seem. The triglycerides in fish oils contain some fifty different fatty acids; those in a vegetable oil like soybean oil contain at least nine. Isolating the saturated fatty acids (stearic and palmitic acid, for example) from these mixtures is a relatively simple procedure since saturated fats have regular, zigzagging carbon chains that stack on, or zipper together, one another, making them a crystal, or solid, even at room temperature.

But polyunsaturated fatty acids were a different matter. Double bonds between carbon atoms introduce sharp bends in the chains of fatty acids, the result of repulsive forces between the hydrogens on those carbons, making crystallization difficult even at extremely low temperatures. It is the difference between stacking logs that are straight and logs with branches sticking out of them, as a chemistry professor once told me. (At least this is how chemists in the 1940s *thought* double bonds acted. More than half a century later, scientists would learn that double bonds can actually make it easier for hydrocarbons to shift rapidly between an uncountable number of positions.)

Increasing the chain length of a fatty acid provides more carbons to be stacked, and with twenty-two carbons in its tail, DHA should crystallize fairly easily. But its six double bonds make crystallization almost impossible. Holman has never seen DHA as a solid, he told me during a visit I made to Austin in 2003. I asked him what that made him think about DHA at the time when he was first trying to purify it, long before the role of DHA in brains and other metabolically active tissues was known. "I don't think I was smart enough to have learned anything from that," he answered. "I was more frustrated than impressed."

Another problem with isolating polyunsaturates is that many of the procedures in a chemist's toolbox (distillation, etc.) cause oxidation of double bonds or affect their location, configuration, or both. The hydrogens on a double bond have a way of flipping from the same side of the molecule (the cis position) to opposite sides (the trans position). Once they are in the trans position, the molecule behaves much more like a saturated fat. It is much more linear and stackable, and so is much more easy to crystallize.

Because of the difficulty of crystallizing polyunsaturates (without changing them in the process), Holman had to find ways of attaching these fatty acids to much larger molecules that could be crystallized, then restoring the fatty acid when he was finished. This was, and is, a laborious procedure with many steps and much loss of material at each one.

It helped to start with fats or oils* that were rich in a particular fatty acid. For linoleic acid, Holman started with cottonseed oil. For alpha linolenic acid, he started with linseed oil; for arachidonic acid, he started with the livers of animals; and for DHA, he followed Burr's advice and went to slaughterhouses to collect the brains of cattle. One cow's brain yielded a small vial of pure DHA, and Holman guarded these glass, vacuum-sealed vials as jealously as a miner does his gold. He built a small travel-

*A word on the use of the terms *fats* and *oils*, and that is that no hard and fast rules apply. *Fats* usually refers to lipids that are solid at room temperature, *oils* to those that are liquid at room temperature. Obvious exceptions are the tropical oils, coconut and palm, that are solid at room temperature despite their name. The animal/vegetable distinction is relevant, too, with animal fats usually referred to as *fats* and vegetable fats as *oils*. But the exception here is fish *oils*. Go figure (or fish). Familiarity also has a great deal to do with what we call these fats. Westerners sometimes call palm oil "tree lard" because this vegetable oil is hard like their familiar cooking fat: lard. Chinese sometimes refer to butter as "cow oil" because they use vegetable oil, never butter, in cooking. I try to stay within accepted usage so as not to confuse readers, but the terms are far from scientific and can be thought of as interchangeable. All fats and oils are triglycerides with an identical backbone (a glycerol molecule) attached to three fatty acids.

ing case for them so that the vials would always remain upright, protected from any impact.

By the end of a year, Holman had enough data for a thesis and had made it possible to study how animals metabolize these fats. He had developed methods for isolating all the unsaturated fatty acids occurring in animal tissues and determining if they had two, three, four, five or six double bonds. Before he went on a postdoctoral fellowship to Stockholm, he and Burr showed that rats who were given different amounts of linoleic and alpha linolenic acid in their diets had different fatty acid profiles in all of their vital organs.

Holman took his forty sealed vials of purified fatty acids with him to Stockholm and to the laboratory of Hugo Theorell at the Karolinska Institute, where he was given the problem of crystallizing an enzyme in soybeans that causes the oxidation of polyunsaturated fatty acids. It was the same sort of reaction that manufacturers of processed food were looking to prevent. Sune Bergström had recently been a graduate student in Theorell's laboratory, and Holman did one small project with this future Nobel Prize winner, long before he revolutionized biology with the information that important cell messengers, known first as prostaglandins and then as eicosanoids, are made out of fatty acids. Holman had nothing to do with that work, but he and his wife, Karla, formed a lasting friendship with the Bergströms.

Holman and his wife planned to spend just one year in Sweden, but they so much enjoyed being in the country, spending time with Holman's Swedish relatives and learning Swedish, that they stayed an extra twelve months. It was an experience "that sweetened their lives" and "made the world their home," Holman told me recently, though the extra year cost him his place at the University of Minnesota.

When Holman returned to the United States, he had to find another position and took a teaching job at the Agricultural and

Mechanical College of Texas (now Texas A&M University). He resumed the feeding experiments he had begun with Burr, and there, on the plains of Texas, as he likes to say, he and a graduate student were the first people to know that feeding rats pure linoleic acid increases the arachidonic acid in their tissues and feeding them pure alpha linolenic acid increases the amount of eicosapentaenoic acid and DHA. They concluded that there are two families of polyunsaturated fatty acids: one derived from the eighteen-carbon linoleic acid (with its two double bonds) and the other from the eighteen-carbon alpha linolenic acid (with its three double bonds).

A very different pattern was seen in the tissues of rats that were fed a fat-free diet. These rats had no arachidonic acid, eicosapentaenoic acid, or DHA in their tissues. But they did have a fatty acid that was derived from the monounsaturated fat oleic acid, the unsaturated fat that animals can make themselves. Holman and his student identified this fat, with its three double bonds, as Mead's acid, a fatty acid recently named for James Mead in California. Mead's acid is found only in fat-deprived animals. It is the best bodies can do—the most unsaturated fatty acid they can make—when they lack both linoleic and alpha linolenic acid.

Holman didn't know why animals prefer a certain amount of polyunsaturated fatty acids in their tissues, but he and a pediatrician, Arild Hansen, began to apply this insight to humans. Hansen had been in medical school at the University of Minnesota when the Burrs ran their unsuccessful experiment on a human volunteer, but he wasn't convinced by the outcome that fats, certain fats, weren't essential for humans. Hansen was aware of the problem of infant eczema that had surfaced in the United States in the 1940s and wondered if the cause was the fats (or the missing fats) in these infants' diets. This was a time when it was common to give infants skim milk and sugar as a substitute for mother's milk.

Hansen began testing babies with severe eczema while he was still at the University of Minnesota. He found that they had lower amounts of polyunsaturated fatty acids in their blood than healthy infants. He also found that he was able to cure many of them by giving them lard, or pork fat, which contains both linoleic and arachidonic acid. The supplements of lard increased the total amount of polyunsaturates in the babies' blood.

Then, when both Hansen and Holman were in Texas in the late 1940s (Holman at Texas A&M and Hansen at the University of Texas Medical School in Galveston), the two scientists continued this work together. They conducted an extensive survey of how infants responded to different formulas and were able to conclude that an infant's requirement for essential fatty acids (which, at the time, meant only linoleic acid) is somewhat greater than 1 percent of its calories. The fat in cow's milk was unable to provide this. Hansen and Holman were also able to show that the best and simplest index of an essential fatty acid deficiency (again, referring only to a deficiency of linoleic acid and its offspring) was the ratio in the blood of Mead's acid (the self-made fatty acid) to arachidonic acid.

Holman took these insights back to Minnesota with him in 1951 when he was offered a position as an associate professor of biochemistry at the Hormel Institute. The institute had recently established a separate home for itself in the stable of the Hormel estate on the east edge of Austin, where one half of the building was devoted to Jay Hormel's cattle, horses, and antique cars, and the other half to three new laboratories and an office. The hayloft was the institute's library, and the "microbiologists had great difficulty keeping things sterile in a laboratory built of rough wood," as Holman remembers in his unpublished autobiography. During this time, the institute became as famous for drinking, card playing, and political infighting as for research, but things settled down in 1958 when modern facilities were built near the Hormel meatpacking plant in Austin itself.

Holman, who served as director of the institute from 1975 to 1985, was never one for card games. Plus, he was on the verge "of his best work ever," as he describes the research he did on his return to Minnesota. Ernst Klenk, a German researcher who had helped Holman learn the techniques of mass spectrometry in 1962, now asked Holman if he had room for one of his graduate students, Hans Mohrhauer. Mohrhauer came to work in Holman's lab, and Holman and this very meticulous German began the experiments that would reveal the fundamental competition between fats. They used all the techniques for separating and analyzing fatty acids that Holman had been inventing and perfecting over the years, as well as the new and more precise methods of gas-liquid chromatography and mass spectrometry. The latter made it possible for chemists to assign a molecular weight to the fats coming off the chromatograph.

Holman already knew that giving rats linoleic acid increased the arachidonic acid in their tissues (and that giving them alpha linolenic acid increased the eicosapentaenoic acid and DHA). Now, he and Mohrhauer gave rats varying amounts, or ratios, of these two parent fats, then monitored their tissues for change.

"It was very confusing at first," remembers Holman. "If you increased the amount of linoleic acid in the diet, the amount of alpha linolenic acid and all the fatty acids derived from alpha linolenic decreased. And vice versa. If you increased the alpha linolenic, the linoleic decreased. And we found this same phenomenon in every tissue of the rat's body." Similarly, when arachidonic acid was fed to the rats as the sole fat in an otherwise fat-free diet, the arachidonic content of tissues increased and the eicosapentaenoic acid and DHA content fell.

Morning in Holman's lab always began with coffee and a quiz from the daily newspaper. Then Holman and his graduate students would talk about these baffling results, proposing one explanation after another, however implausible. The explanation that Holman ultimately chose, the one that best suited the results and has been substantiated by decades of research in laboratories around the world, was that they were observing "a competitive affair between the families of polyunsaturated fatty acids. We realized that linoleic acid and linolenic acid must be metabolized by the same set of enzymes, and that they were competing with each other at each step of the desaturation and elongation process," says Holman. "As we increased one family in the diet, we suppressed the metabolism of the other."

The concept of competition between fatty acids was not entirely new. James Mead had already published evidence that high levels of oleic acid, a monounsaturated fat, in the diet of guinea pigs suppresses the metabolism of linoleic acid, producing symptoms of hair loss and poor growth similar to those that the Burrs had observed in their fat-deprived rats.

But Holman expanded this concept to include the family of polyunsaturated fatty acids based on alpha linolenic acid, a family that few people then thought important. Interestingly, alpha linolenic acid is a much better competitor than linoleic acid, since smaller amounts of it are able to suppress the metabolic products of the other. That competitive edge is easily overwhelmed, as Holman and Mohrhauer found, by large amounts of linoleic acid. Similarly, both alpha linolenic and linoleic acids are better competitors than oleic acid, but their edge can be overwhelmed by large amounts of saturated fats or oleic acid in the diet. Oleic acid is made from the saturated fat palmitic acid by a two-carbon elongation and the introduction of one double bond. It is the main fatty acid in olive oil, remember, and the one unsaturated fatty acid we can make from scratch.

Holman began writing up these interesting interactions as an invited paper in the Swedish medical journal *Acta Chemica Scandinavica*. The paper would be published in a special supplement in honor of his former professor in Sweden, Hugo Theorell, who had won the 1955 Nobel Prize in Medicine for his work with oxidation enzymes, including lipoxygenase, the enzyme that Holman had successfully crystallized during his time at the Karolinska Institute. As Holman was writing, he struggled with a way to describe the relationships between the different families of fatty acids.

Nomenclature in chemistry begins with the highest-priority group of a molecule, which in lipids is the most charged or polar group, the carboxylic acid. But if Holman started with the acidic end of the fatty acids, their names would change with each step of elongation and desaturation. No one would be able to see the relationships between them. For example, alpha linolenic acid, with a chemical name of 9,12,15-octadecatrienoic acid, would become 5,8,11,14,17-eicosapentaenoic acid with the addition of two carbons and two double bonds, and 4,7,10,13,16,19-docosahexaenoic acid, DHA, with the addition of two more carbons and a double bond. Linoleic acid, with a chemical name of 9,12-octadecadienoic acid, would become 6,9,12-octadecatrienoic acid, dihomo-gamma-linolenic acid, with the addition of one double bond, and 5,8,11,14-eicosatetraenoate, arachidonic acid, with the addition of two carbons and one more double bond. Abbreviations of the Geneva nomenclature, according to which linoleic acid is 9,12–18:2 and arachidonic acid is 5,8,11,1–20:4, also do not show the close relationships between these two, or any other, fatty acids.

"It takes study!" Holman says. "Which made writing about these interactions almost impossible to follow. I had to have something to shorten things up and to show relativity so you didn't have to ponder those relationships." As he wrestled with this problem, Holman thought about something that Klenk had first mentioned to him in the 1950s: the tails of the polyunsaturated fatty acids remained the same throughout all the steps of elongation and desaturation. In other words, if you go to the last carbon and count backward, all the members of one family have their first double bonds three carbons from the end. All the members of the second family have their first double bond six carbons from the end. And all the members of the third family, the family we can make from start to finish, have their first double bond nine carbons in.

Chemists frequently use the first letters of the Greek alphabet—alpha, beta, and gamma—to indicate the position of chemical groups, as Holman knew. And from the many years he had spent in a Baptist Sunday school and his familiarity with the book of Revelation, he knew that omega, ω, was the last letter of the Greek alphabet. So Holman had the idea of naming the families of polyunsaturated fatty acids by the part that distinguishes them the most, their tails or ends—the part, Holman says, while wiggling his fingers, "that's in contact with the outside world."

"Things were changing everywhere but at the end of the molecule," the chemist adds. "We had to consider that the end must have a function."

Turning his attention to the end of these fatty acids, Holman found that he could describe them with many fewer characters. The whole structure of linoleic acid could be described by using only six characters: 18:2ω6. The whole structure of alpha linolenic acid could be described by 18:3ω3. Plus, this new terminology made it easy to distinguish alpha linolenic acid from other linolenic acids, those derived from linoleic acid. The latter would be 20:3ω6 and 18:3ω6. Oleic acid could be quickly described as 18:1ω9 and Mead's acid as 20:3ω9.

Holman and Mohrhauer introduced this new nomenclature in their paper in the Swedish journal without any fanfare; they put 22:5ω6 in parentheses after the chemical name of the molecule it described (4,7,10,13,16-docosapentaenoate), followed by asterisks that led to a note at the bottom of the page. There readers found an explanation: "This shorthand formula indicates 22 carbon atoms and 5 double bonds, the nearest of which lies 6 carbon atoms from the terminal methyl group. This notation is necessary to avoid confusion between isomeric metabolites of oleate, linoleate and linolenate."

Holman might have first used this notation "to avoid confusion" between isomers, molecules with different arrangements of the same number of atoms. But he realized almost immediately how handy this new notation was in creating family trees. In a footnote to a paper in the *Journal of Lipid Research*, published the next year, in 1964, Holman writes, "To avoid confusion between isomers and to point out family relationships, acids having the first double bond between the third and fourth carbon atoms from the terminal methyl group are designated ω3 and are related to linolenate. Those related to linoleate are designated ω6 and those related to oleate, ω9."

I asked Holman how the scientific community had reacted to this innovative terminology. We were sitting in the living room of his modest house in Austin, surrounded by furniture Holman had made and photographs of his late wife, Karla, and of the orchids he used to grow as a hobby. "At first, scientists didn't think there was a need for it," he said. "Then, for a while, it looked as if it might disappear, especially when some other scientists tried to replace it with an n system." These were scientists, he added mischievously, "who hadn't been to Sunday school."

OMEGA-3 FAMILY TREE

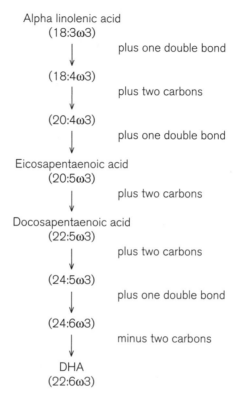

Alpha linolenic acid
(18:3ω3)
↓ plus one double bond

(18:4ω3)
↓ plus two carbons

(20:4ω3)
↓ plus one double bond

Eicosapentaenoic acid
(20:5ω3)
↓ plus two carbons

Docosapentaenoic acid
(22:5ω3)
↓ plus two carbons

(24:5ω3)
↓ plus one double bond

(24:6ω3)
↓ minus two carbons

DHA
(22:6ω3)

FIGURE 2 Omega-3 family tree. Only the named members of the omega-3 family accumulate in tissues in any significant amount. The rest are short-lived intermediates. Eicosapentaenoic acid and DHA are the principal metabolites of alpha linolenic acid; they are interconverted through docosapentaenoic acid.

OMEGA-6 FAMILY TREE

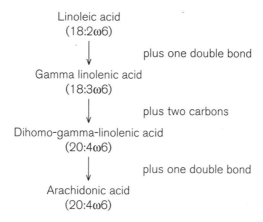

Linoleic acid
(18:2ω6)

plus one double bond

Gamma linolenic acid
(18:3ω6)

plus two carbons

Dihomo-gamma-linolenic acid
(20:4ω6)

plus one double bond

Arachidonic acid
(20:4ω6)

FIGURE 3 Omega-6 family tree. In healthy, well-nourished individuals, the omega-6 family tree usually ends with arachidonic acid. When much more linoleic acid than alpha linolenic acid is consumed, enzymes turn arachidonic acid into 22:4ω6 and, finally, 22:5ω6 (adrenic and docosapentaenoic acid), its illegitimate children, one might say

"But something about *omega* rolls off the tongue easily," Holman went on. "I couldn't see it coming, but all of a sudden *omegas* has become a common word." In retrospect, Holman thinks he should have introduced his new nomenclature in a bigger way, by publishing it in an American journal, which would have attracted more readers. But he's gratified to know that the vocabulary he invented four decades ago is finally catching on—in tandem, it seems, with the growing awareness of the importance of omega-3s.

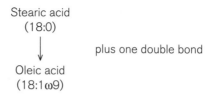

OMEGA-9 FAMILY TREE

FIGURE 4 Omega-9 family tree. In the absence of omega-6s and omega-3s, enzymes turn oleic acid into 18:2ω9, then 20:2ω9, and finally 20:3ω9, or Mead's acid.

And perhaps the omega vocabulary wasn't necessary in 1963, when the only fats that were even suspected of being essential to humans were linoleic acid and its derivatives. But it has become necessary as we have come to know the omega-3s and as scientists—and the public—have needed to distinguish between the different families of polyunsaturated fats.

Today's scientists tend to shy away from the omega nomenclature precisely because it is popular with the public. They prefer the *n-x* system in which *n* represents the number of carbons in a fatty acid and *x* is the number of carbons from the end where the last double bond is located. (By this convention, linoleic acid is 18:2n-6 and the family of fatty acids based on linoleic acid is the n-6 family.) This system works, but it isn't as good as the omega system because "it doesn't immediately send you to the end of the molecule," as Holman points out. And it doesn't, of course, give Holman his due.

The first time Holman saw his nomenclature being used, at a local grocery store several years ago, he was so excited that he rushed back home to get his camera. He returned to the store to photograph the sign at the fish counter: "Omega-3s are here."

FOUR

MONSIEUR CHOLESTEROL

A man is only as old as his arteries.

DR. WILLIAM OSLER, 1892

RALPH HOLMAN WASN'T INTERESTED IN CHOLESTEROL WHEN HE WAS looking for a new research project in 1941. But there was someone at the University of Minnesota who would be taken by this waxy substance, the stuff of plaques, as well as normal tissues, hormones, and vitamins. That was Ancel Keys, the charismatic physiologist who turned cholesterol into a household name and who even earned the nickname "Monsieur Cholesterol" because of his decades of work linking fat in the diet to elevated levels of cholesterol in the blood.

"Keys had a beneficial effect because he focused people's attention on lipids," says Holman, who had known Keys since the physiologist sat on his dissertation committee. "But he was dogmatic about the part fats played in heart disease long before the nature of different fats was understood. Everywhere I went with my essential fatty acids, he went with his serum cholesterol. I couldn't compete in terms of personality, but I could compete in terms of data."

Keys established a seemingly irrefutable link between fat consumption and heart disease. But ever since his first pronouncements in the 1950s, the guilty fats—all fats, saturated fats, animal fats, tropical fats, cholesterol, trans fats—have kept changing as research has revealed how the different fats behave. Some people have been tolerant of these frequent changes. Others have become so frustrated that they have thrown the baby out with the bathwater and rejected all advice about fat.

The baby, in this case, is the importance of diet and exercise in the prevention of heart disease, a point that Keys, inarguably, was one of the first to make. It's hard to imagine there was ever a time when diet wasn't thought of as a risk factor for heart disease, but Keys appreciated this connection long before most other scientists and physicians. Americans have Sunday dinner every day, he told *Time* magazine in 1959. In the late 1950s, he spearheaded the large and influential Seven Countries Study to follow the health and diets of 12,763 men in Yugoslavia, Finland, Italy, the Netherlands, Greece, the United States, and Japan.

After earning his Ph.D. in physiology from the University of Cambridge in England, Keys taught at Harvard for several years; then, in 1940, he came to Minnesota to found the Laboratory of Physiological Hygiene. This laboratory, which was located underneath the University of Minnesota's Memorial Stadium, Gate 27, quickly became a center for research in nutrition, preventive medicine, and epidemiology. At the beginning of the Second World War, Keys served as a special assistant to the secretary of war and was in charge of developing the eponymous K ration, which started out, he once said, as little more than a bag lunch.

Toward the end of the war, it became clear to Keys that starvation would be a major problem in occupied countries such as Holland and Norway, and he began researching the effects of prolonged food deprivation. He reduced the caloric intake of thirty-six conscientious objectors (males who had volunteered for the project as a form of alternative service) to half the normal intake for six months. Predictably, these men lost much of their body weight and became food obsessed. Three months after the Minnesota Starvation Experiment ended, none had regained his former weight or physical capacity. Keys learned that effective rehabilitation requires that starved individuals take in far more calories than normal for several months, as well as vitamin supplements and a higher proportion of protein in their diet, all of which he recommended to national and international relief agencies. "Starved people cannot be taught democracy," the physiologist observed later. "To talk about the will of the people when you aren't feeding them is perfect hogwash."

As Keys had predicted, some populations in war-torn Europe suffered from starvation. But others experienced a positive benefit from the conflict that no one had foreseen. Health professionals in Finland, Sweden, Norway, and Holland all observed and reported on a sudden drop in the number of people dying from heart disease, the condition that the doctors in the different countries variously diagnosed as angina pectoris, myocardial infarction, chronic myocarditis, arteriosclerosis, myocardial degeneration, pericarditis, emboli, and thrombosis. This steep decline in deaths occurred even in areas where food shortages were not acute. And it affected all ages of the population, though its impact on the youngest groups tended to be the greatest.

After the war, after food supplies had been restored, the death rate from heart disease began to rise again, as steeply and rapidly as it had fallen, giving health professionals a window onto this condition, a plague of modern Western life that had become the most common cause of death. Before the war, the rise in heart disease since the turn of the century had been seen as an inevitable consequence of an extended life span: the result of older populations facing fewer causes of death. The war experience greatly weakened this explanation.

In the years before the war, rises in heart disease had also been attributed to rising levels of stress in increasingly urbanized populations. But if that were the case, then surely the disease would have ravaged the war-torn, displaced populations. The sharp decline in deaths during the war, especially among young people, turned scientists' attention away from stress and aging populations and toward diet—in particular, toward the foods that were in short supply during the war: meats, butter, cheeses, and eggs.

To be sure, some earlier reports linking the diets of populations to their incidence of heart disease had appeared in the literature. But these had attracted little notice, because the populations that were being compared—the Indonesians and the Dutch, for instance, in the work of the Dutch physician C. D. de Langen—differed from each other in so many ways. Trying to pinpoint *the* difference responsible for heart disease was like looking for the proverbial needle in a haystack. During the Second World War, though, the same populations acted as their own controls, and many researchers, including Ancel Keys, were understandably intrigued.

When Keys first heard about this curious downturn in deaths, he began examining the incidence of heart disease in different countries (as best he could, given the discrepancies in systems of diagnosis and record keeping) and concluded that the rates did indeed vary. The rate for the United States, for example, was far worse than for Italy or Portugal. He then devised studies to determine which foods might be responsible for these trends, using a food's ability to raise the cholesterol in an individual's blood as a marker for its tendency to promote heart disease. Serum cholesterol, in the 1940s and early '50s, was the only known risk factor for heart disease, and it was the only thing for which there was a test. Keys therefore put schizophrenics at the

Hastings State Hospital on six different diets to see what foods would raise and lower the cholesterol in their blood. He fed egg yolks to St. Paul businessmen to see if dietary cholesterol, present in high concentration in egg yolks, was as dangerous as some people thought.

Dietary cholesterol had been suspected of causing heart disease as early as 1913, long before heart disease had become a public health problem, when scientists in Russia fed pure cholesterol to rabbits and observed the rapid onset of lesions resembling plaques in human patients with atherosclerosis. Moreover, as I've already mentioned, cholesterol is one of the main components of plaques. It seemed only logical that cholesterol in the diet would lead to cholesterol in the arteries.

But Keys's experiments with feeding cholesterol to humans produced very little effect on their serum cholesterol, and he concluded that the attempt to extrapolate from experiments with rabbits "can lead to absurdities." These animals "have little or no dietary experience with cholesterol after weaning," he explained, "and have little capacity to destroy or otherwise eliminate it when they are fed large amounts."

Dietary fat, on the other hand, had a pronounced effect on the serum cholesterol of these schizophrenics and businessmen, and fat became Keys's target throughout his long career of fighting heart disease. Keys researched the fat content of the diets of different countries and published a chart in 1953 showing an almost perfect linear correlation between the number of deaths from heart disease and the percentage of calories consumed as fat. He included six countries in this chart—Japan, Italy, England, Australia, Canada, and the United States. The percentage of calories consumed as fat ranged from less than 10 percent, in Japan, to close to 40 percent, in the United States. The incidence of heart disease ranged from fewer than 100 deaths per hundred thousand inhabitants to 700.

The chart created a stir, especially after President Eisenhower's heart attack in 1955. And though a few scientists criticized Keys for including just six countries, not the twenty-two countries for which data existed, his message quickly caught on. It helped that Keys was a forceful speaker with a definite answer and none of the doubts and reservations of other researchers. Perhaps it also helped that he never lost the English accent he had acquired during his years at Cambridge and that some people, Holman included, thought that this California-born scientist was in fact English.

(If all twenty-two countries for which data existed were included, the graph relating fat consumption to deaths from heart disease looked like "buckshot hitting a page instead of a straight line," as one researcher puts it. The scatter of points suggested some association between the two variables, the authors of a critical paper concluded. "But the selection of the original six countries, for whatever reason, greatly exaggerated its importance." As it should have, for the quality of fat and the balance between the different families of fats, as we now know, are more important than the quantity.)

According to Keys's original thesis, the only thing that mattered in the link between fat and heart disease was the quantity of fat consumed. At first, Keys didn't even distinguish between the effects of saturated and unsaturated fats, though Ed Ahrens at the Rockefeller Institute had been reporting on significant differences between the two since the early 1950s. At a conference in 1957, when a young scientist pointed out that unsaturated fats don't raise serum cholesterol nearly as much as saturated fats do, Keys tried to shoot him down. "Saturated, unsaturated," he remembers Keys saying. "I don't think you understand this field, young man." (The scientist asked to remain unnamed because the story might sound like "sour grapes.")

Soon after, Keys did acknowledge the research of Ed Ahrens. But he confused the growing understanding of what it is about polyunsaturated fats that is important (their linoleic acid content, as some thought, or their degree of unsaturation) with his dismissal of the benefits of fish oil. "The fish industry is heartened by imaginative statements that coronary heart-disease is absent in Eskimos and rare in Norwegians because of their consumption of marine oils," as he wrote in 1957.

Keys was also forced to amend his original thesis to acknowledge that dietary cholesterol has a small but significant effect on serum cholesterol and that the monounsaturated fats in olive oil are not neutral, as he first contended. For whatever reasons, physicians and health professionals followed loyally in the wake of these amendments. When Keys began to distinguish between saturated and unsaturated fats, the world divided fats into two camps, animal and vegetable, failing to recognize that no fat is totally saturated or unsaturated and that some of the most saturated fats—coconut and palm oil—are derived from plant sources. When he acknowledged the positive effect of monounsaturated fats, he was taken up by olive oil companies and left Minnesota to work, then retire, in Italy.

Keys was not the first researcher to link serum cholesterol to heart disease, but he popularized the association to such an extent that the two became synonymous in the public's mind. Good fats were those that lowered serum cholesterol, and bad fats were those that raised it—a message that obscured important truths and unknowns. Among them were the facts that fats do more than just raise and lower serum cholesterol and that cholesterol does more than just hang around the blood. Of the cholesterol in the body, only a small amount, 5 percent, is found in the blood. The rest is located in membranes (including the membranes of brain cells), hormones, vitamins, bile acids, and so on, where it is critical to normal functioning.

Also lost was a truth about serum cholesterol: it was, is, and always will be nothing more than a surrogate marker for heart disease. No one has ever demonstrated how elevated levels of this fat in the blood actually cause heart disease. Half the people with heart disease don't have elevated cholesterol levels. Half the people with elevated cholesterol don't have heart disease. The idea had gradually taken hold that high serum cholesterol leads to heart disease through a slow accumulation of fatty plaques in the arteries, causing a blockage in the supply of blood to the heart and a tendency for blood to clot. There was little proof for this mechanism, though, and researchers would later learn that most thrombosis, or clotting, occurs in arteries that are not blocked by plaque.

Lost as well in all of Keys's staunch assertiveness was the reality of what fats people were actually eating when the incidence of heart disease began to soar. By the 1960s, Keys had come to blame saturated fats for the rise in heart disease since the turn of the century. But the intake of saturated fats had, in fact, been declining in the United States during this time—from 42 percent of fat calories to 34 percent. The intake of calories from linoleic acid, on the other hand, had been steadily increasing—from 7 percent of the total fat intake in 1909–13 to about 13 percent in 1967—partly in response to recommendations to substitute vegetable oils and margarine for butter and lard.

Scientists were correct in reporting that polyunsaturated oils and margarine lower serum cholesterol, and that they lack dietary cholesterol (which had come in the public's mind to be thoroughly and mistakenly entwined with serum cholesterol). But more recent research has shown that a high consumption of linoleic acid, the most prevalent polyunsaturate in many vegetable oils, is associated with many other risk factors for heart disease, including an increase in blood pressure, inflammation, and the tendency of platelets to aggregate.

The certainty surrounding Keys's lipid hypothesis also obscured one of the most interesting features of the fall and rise of heart disease observed during the war: both were precipitous, which should have called into question the notion that heart disease arises from a slow and gradual accumulation of plaque in the arteries. In Norway, mortality from heart disease showed a rising tendency up to the year 1941 (to more than 300 deaths per one hundred thousand inhabitants), before falling steeply in 1941, the first "lean" year of the war (to a low of fewer than 240 deaths). It started climbing back up in 1945.

Meanwhile, the rate in America was steadily climbing. Clearly, something else was going on in the citizens of Norway besides a pause, or interruption, in their gradual accumulation of plaque. A new model of the cause of heart disease was necessary, but it would have to wait until the work of Bang and Dyerberg began raising questions about the old one. Only then would researchers revisit the dietary changes that had occurred during the Second World War. Only then would they appreciate that a decline in the consumption of meats, butter, cheese, and eggs had not been the only change in diet during the war. There had been a simultaneous increase in the consumption of a number of other foods, including cereals, potatoes, vegetables—and fish.

FIVE

FISHY FATS

A bend in the stalk can be seen, but not a bend in the heart.

MAORI SAYING

DYERBERG AND BANG HAD NO IDEA THAT THEIR WORK WOULD UPSET the apple cart of Keys's model. Not after their first trip to Greenland in 1970. Not even after Dyerberg visited Ralph Holman in Minnesota and learned the name of the fatty acid that was so prevalent in the red blood cells of Eskimos.

Eicosapentaenoic acid was, after all, a polyunsaturated fatty acid; and polyunsaturates, as Keys had come to acknowledge, lower the cholesterol in an individual's blood. The presence of high levels of eicosapentaenoic acid in the Eskimos' blood would nicely explain why their serum cholesterol was low despite their high intake of fat and cholesterol. And their low serum cholesterol would explain their low rate of heart disease in terms of the classic model, which depicts cholesterol as accumulating in blood vessels and eventually reducing blood flow to the heart.

But on Dyerberg and Bang's second trip to Greenland, in 1972, a trip on which they hoped to show that the unusual fats in the Eskimos' blood did indeed come from the fats in their unusual diet, the two Danish physicians made the mistake of freeze-drying their food samples (instead of deep-freezing them or freeze-drying them under nitrogen), thereby exposing them to oxygen under low pressure and destroying many of their unsaturated fatty acids. The incorrect values they got when they ran those freeze-dried samples on their gas-liquid chromatograph contradicted Keys's theory and equations and opened their minds to new ideas about the mechanisms and causes of heart disease. It was a fortunate error; by the time they realized their mistake and returned to Greenland to collect new samples, in 1976, they were well on their way to initiating a coup.

Not that it was immediately recognized as such. In the United States, in 1976, the prevailing opinion was that "nutrition science has developed essentially all the basic knowledge that is necessary" to determine what people should be eating in order to reduce their risk of diet-related cancers and heart disease, as Dr. Gio Gori of the National Institute of Cancer told the U.S. Senate's Committee on Nutrition and Human Needs, which was chaired by George McGovern. Linoleic acid had been accepted as an essential nutrient for humans in the 1960s. But very few people were suggesting that alpha linolenic acid, or any other member of the omega-3 family, might be essential as well.

In 1984, six years after Dyerberg, Bang, and their collaborators in England published a paradigm-altering paper in *Lancet*— "Eicosapentaenoic Acid and Prevention of Thrombosis and Atherosclerosis?"—the National Institutes of Health (NIH) published its *Consensus Development Conference Statement* on cholesterol, advising Americans that the most effective way to prevent heart disease was to reduce their intake of dietary cholesterol and other fats. The scientists who signed on to this infamous consensus statement ("infamous" because dissenting researchers point out that the conclusions were anything but a consensus) seemed unaware that a family of important nutrients was in the process of being recognized as essential. And that these nutrients not only are fats themselves but have a profound influence on the way that other fats, cholesterol included, are moved around the body.

Dyerberg and Bang's second trip to Greenland took place during the summer of 1972, the same time of year as their previous trip.

Gas-liquid chromatography was still fairly new, and there were only a few reports on the fatty acid content of different foods. But it was known that fish, especially cold-water fish like salmon, were full of polyunsaturates. The two Danish researchers wanted to know if this was true for whale and seal meat as well—and whether those polyunsaturates included eicosapentaenoic acid.

So Bang and Dyerberg returned to one of the communities they had visited before, Igdlorssuit (literally, "the place of big houses," though its dwellings were only slightly more commodious than those in nearby settlements), and asked seven of the people who had participated in their earlier study to provide them with duplicate amounts of all the foods they ate during one week. The researchers would, of course, pay them for these foods and for their trouble, negotiating the price with each participant over coffee. After receiving these weekly meal plans of seal, whale, and fish, as well as the small amounts of rice, potatoes, and sugar that participants had purchased from the one-room trading store in the settlement, Bang and Dyerberg homogenized them, then took samples from the slurries for freeze-drying and analysis in Denmark.

There, they weren't surprised to find that the carbohydrate content of the Eskimo diet was less than that of the typical Dane (37 percent of calories versus 47), nor that the cholesterol content of the Eskimo diet was much higher than that of Danes (245 milligrams of cholesterol for every thousand calories versus 139). But they were intrigued that the total fat content of the two diets was very similar (37 percent of calories for the Eskimos and 42 percent for the Danes) and expected that the explanation for the Eskimos' low serum cholesterol and low rate of heart disease, despite this similarity in fat intake, would be a high intake of polyunsaturates. Much of the fat in the Danish diet comes from pork and dairy products—the Danes were known at the time for buttering their cheese as well as their bread—and is very saturated.

Keys had published a formula in 1965 that was supposed to give the difference in the serum cholesterol one could expect between two populations with different fat contents in their diets. I include it here to show the source of Dyerberg and Bang's confusion—and how precise Keys's ideas were: "The difference in the mean serum cholesterol of two populations = $2.7(\Delta S - \Delta 1/2P) + 1.5(\sqrt{C_2} - \sqrt{C_1})$, where S and P are the percentages of calories from saturated and unsaturated fats, and C_1 and C_2 are the cholesterol content of the two diets." The Danish physicians thought the numbers from their Eskimo data would support this formula, as I said. But because of the mistake with freeze-drying, they didn't. When Bang and Dyerberg plugged all their numbers into Keys's equation, the mean serum cholesterol of the Eskimos should have been just 8 milligrams or so below that of the Danes—not the 40 milligrams it actually was.

Bang and Dyerberg concluded that DHA and eicosapentaenoic acid, two polyunsaturates that they had found in greater abundance in Eskimo than in Danish foods, "may be of major importance for the rather low serum cholesterol levels in Eskimos," and that their action on serum cholesterol (and on all the other lipid fractions: triglycerides, LDLs, and VLDLs) "may differ qualitatively" from that of other polyunsaturated fatty acids.

The Danish physicians learned of their mistake with the freeze-drying only by chance, when Robert Ackman, the Canadian fish biologist who had developed many of the first techniques for analyzing fish oils, contacted them about an unrelated matter. They immediately began planning a third trip to Greenland to collect new samples. They didn't want to make any mistakes this time, so they got in touch with someone they thought could help them: Hugh Sinclair, an English researcher who had once collected food samples in northern Canada. Sinclair was also very interested in essential fatty acids and the role of fats in health and diet, but Bang and Dyerberg didn't know that at the time. Nor did they know of Sinclair's reputation as an eccentric and scientific gadfly.

Sinclair had been interested in the subject of fats ever since visiting the lab of George Burr's professor, Harold Evans, in the 1930s, and he had published a very controversial letter in the *Lancet* in 1956, suggesting that atherosclerosis, and many other diseases of Western countries, was caused by a chronic deficiency of essential fatty acids. By this he meant all the omega-6s and the omega-3s.

Today, you will hear it said that Sinclair was on the right track about heart disease and years ahead of his time, even prophetic. And he was indeed ahead of his time in thinking of all the polyunsaturates as essential fatty acids. But he was so fundamentally wrong about Western diets being deficient in linoleic acid and was so unscientific in his language and methods that he made it disreputable to talk about essential fatty acids and heart disease in the same breath. Hans Krebs, the 1953 Nobel Prize winner in medicine, is said to have taken a sledgehammer to Sinclair's lab after the *Lancet* letter, and Sinclair's funding and reputation suffered greatly.

Bang and Dyerberg didn't know anything about this history, though, when they visited the elderly scientist in his large, rambling house in a small village near Reading. When he surprised them by asking if he could join them on the trip to Greenland, they quickly agreed. They were a little concerned because the trip would be in the winter this time, by dogsled, and Sinclair was in his seventies. But they were won over by the enthusiasm of "this fine old gentleman," as they saw him at first, with his penchant for interjecting scientific papers with verse.

> In Hudson Bay, far far away
> From Simpson's choicest torso,

went the limerick in Sinclair's paper on the diet of Canadian Eskimos, the paper that brought him to the attention of Dyerberg and Bang;

> You can get a meal from an Elephant seal
> As pleasant if not more so.
>
> Anonymous

Sinclair did more talking than science on the 1976 trip to Igdlorssuit. Dyerberg says that he and Bang would "always end up learning which nobleman and prince of Arabia he knew," a steady stream of information that was "fun for about a half an hour." But even without his help, the two Danes collected all the samples they needed and returned to Denmark to generate a new set of data that jibed almost perfectly with Keys's equation.

This could have been the end of the Greenland story. Bang and Dyerberg could have concluded that all was right with Keys's model and that all the polyunsaturates protect equally against heart disease. But during the interval, in the time when Dyerberg and Bang were thinking that there was something unusual about the polyunsaturates the Eskimos consumed (eicosapentaenoic acid, especially), they were doing a great deal of reading about fats. Some of the papers they read had to do with the potent cell messengers called prostaglandins that were made from twenty-carbon fatty acids.

Prostaglandins were first discovered in the 1930s by physicians who were experimenting with artificial insemination and found that a compound in semen sometimes produces a violent contraction of the uterus. At first, prostaglandins were thought to be produced only by male reproductive tissues (thus their name, from the prostate gland). But in the 1960s, Sune Bergström, Ralph Holman's friend from Sweden, discovered that many different types of tissues produce prostaglandin-like compounds and that these compounds cause a wide array of reactions, from muscle contractions and inflammation to rapid changes in blood pressure.

Bergström was also one of the scientists to report, in 1964, that prostaglandins were made from twenty-carbon fatty acids. He suspected this to be the case because of the location and kind of double bonds (cis rather than trans bonds) in both, but he needed fatty acids with a radioactive label or tag in order to prove it. He therefore called Dr. David van Dorp at Unilever in Holland to ask if van Dorp could supply him with the necessary compounds. "Are you thinking about what I'm thinking about?" Bergström remembers van Dorp asking. "I only had to say yes," Bergström wrote in an account of this consequential telephone call. Van Dorp supplied Bergström with what he needed. Within weeks, both groups had found that the incubation of labeled fatty acids with sheep testicles yielded large amounts of labeled prostaglandins. They published their findings in the same issue of *Biochimica et Biophysica Acta*.

Prostaglandins, later to be given the less confusing name of *eicosanoids* (from *eikosi*—again, the Greek word for twenty), behave in the manner of fast-acting, short-lived, hormone-like compounds, as Bergström showed, and deliver messages between cells and tissues in localized areas. They caught Bang and Dyerberg's attention only after their story began to come together with that of heart disease.

This convergence began in the early 1970s, when two other researchers at the Karolinska Institute, Mats Hamberg and Bengt Samuelsson (a student of Bergström's), identified a prostaglandin produced by the platelets in blood. The new substance caused platelets to aggregate, or clump together, so they called it *thromboxane*, because platelet aggregation is the first step of thrombosis or blood clotting. Once platelets clump together, they cause the growth of a threadlike net, which traps red blood cells and stops blood flow.

Thromboxane is a very unstable substance, with a half-life of only about 32 seconds in an aqueous environment. It causes a rapid aggregation of platelets and then quickly decomposes. The same substance, it turned out, had previously been detected by the pharmacologist John Vane in England. But he had called this potent compound *rabbit aorta contracting substance* because it also constricts blood vessels.

John Vane, later to become Sir John Vane for the Nobel Prize that he, Bergström, and Samuelsson would win for this work, had already made the important finding that aspirin and aspirin-like substances, the most widely used medicines in the world, produce their effects by blocking the production of prostaglandins. They inhibit the enzyme that converts twenty-carbon fatty acids into substances like thromboxane, the cyclooxygenase (or COX) enzyme. Now, Vane was about to fill out the picture of how prostaglandins affect blood flow with his discovery, in 1976, of a new member of this family of compounds with the opposite effect of thromboxane. This new compound, which he called *prostacyclin*, is made not by platelets, as is thromboxane, but by the cells that line the blood vessels. Those cells release it when incited by platelets or some other stimulus, and it counters the action of thromboxane. It acts to reduce aggregation and clotting.

Suddenly, everyone was talking about prostacyclin and thromboxane, and how the seemingly simple act of blood flowing through blood vessels was a complex interplay between the forces of aggregation and anti-aggregation—a yin-yang, push-me-pull-you dynamic between compounds released by the platelets and compounds released by the vessel walls.

Like other scientists all around the world, Bang and Dyerberg were aware of the developments taking place in prostaglandin research. They were aware of all the attention being given to arachidonic acid because it is a precursor of both thromboxane and prostacyclin and helps make both blood flow and blood clotting possible. In 1976, they were reading a paper out of Vane's laboratory when they remembered the curious finding from their first trip to Greenland: the high arachidonic acid levels in the blood of Danes and the high eicosapentaenoic acid levels in the blood of Eskimos. In the lab one day, one turned to the other and asked, "What if eicosapentaenoic acid could be used to make a different form of thromboxane and prostacyclin?" This process might produce a new balance between the forces that work for and against clotting in a person's blood and might explain why the Eskimos, who have so much eicosapentaenoic acid in their blood and tissues, have so few heart attacks.

At least that was the story Dyerberg and Bang told for many years. In my interview with Dyerberg, he made it clear that the idea had been his, but that the two of them later agreed to say it had occurred to both simultaneously. It was a good idea, whoever had it, and the two doctors immediately tested it by taking blood from a volunteer, then adding equal amounts of either arachidonic or eicosapentaenoic acid. The arachidonic acid caused the platelets in the blood to clump together, as they knew it would.

When they added eicosapentaenoic acid, the reaction was much subdued.

Soon after this promising finding, Dyerberg was scheduled to attend a meeting in England, and from his hotel room in London he made one of the most important telephone calls of his life— to John Vane at the Wellcome Research Laboratories in Kent. Dyerberg introduced himself and began by telling Vane how much he admired him. Then he started talking about the Eskimos. At one point in his story, Dyerberg paused, and Vane said to him, "Talk on. Talk on." When Dyerberg finished, Vane asked, "Jørn, where are you? I'll send a car for you." Dyerberg recalls being very happy that Vane remembered his name.

The idea that a less-aggregating form of thromboxane could be made out of eicosapentaenoic acid was obviously intriguing to Vane. Nor would he have seen it as far-fetched. Dyerberg and Bang may not have known it, but the prostaglandins identified by Sune Bergström in the late 1950s and early '60s (PgE and PgF) were known to exist in three different forms depending on whether their starting material was arachidonic acid, eicosapentaenoic acid, or dihomo-gamma-linolenic acid, a third twenty-carbon fatty acid that is an omega-6 fatty acid and the immediate precursor of arachidonic acid. The prostaglandins made from arachidonic acid got the most attention because they were always the most potent compounds, as well as the most abundant, and because arachidonic acid had been suspected of being an essential fatty acid ever since the Burrs' experiments in the 1930s. But Vane would have known that eicosapentaenoic acid was a possible precursor for the newly discovered thromboxane and prostacyclin. The Eskimos' low rate of heart disease spelled out the enormous health implications of this idea.

Dyerberg recalls that at their first meeting in Kent, Vane outlined the experiments he thought they should do and invited

Dyerberg to come back and "do some research together and then we'll apply for a patent of EPA." They never received that patent, because eicosapentaenoic acid is a natural compound and cannot be patented, but the experiments were a success, leading to a paper in the *Lancet* in 1978. There, they showed that platelets can indeed use eicosapentaenoic acid to make a different and less-aggregating form of thromboxane and that the endothelial cells of blood vessels can use it to make a form of prostacyclin that is almost as anti-aggregating as that made from arachidonic acid. A large amount of eicosapentaenoic acid in the diet would clearly shift the balance in a person's blood vessels away from aggregation. The paper ended with the suggestion that eicosapentaenoic acid "may reduce the development of thrombosis and atherosclerosis in the Western World" and led, as Dyerberg remembers, to discussion of the benefits of fish oil at "each and every cocktail party."

The paper also produced the first of many backlashes from the food industry, because it pointed out that the fats in margarines might not be the most beneficial for health. Margarines are full of polyunsaturates, but those polyunsaturates are largely linoleic acid—the parent of arachidonic acid, the fatty acid from which the most potent and aggregating prostaglandins are formed. Everyone knew this before the *Lancet* paper, but before then, no one thought there was anything anyone could do about it. Arachidonic acid was a given. It was made from linoleic acid, and linoleic acid was essential for health. One had to take the good with the bad.

Dyerberg was stunned when, having been invited to the Netherlands to visit Unilever, one of the world's largest food manufacturers and the producer of the then popular Blue Band margarine, he was subjected to hours of "cruel and tough" questioning. A 1979 letter to the *Lancet* from three Unilever researchers raised questions about the safety of the "n-3" fatty acids, suggesting that they might actually cause the death of heart tissues and be responsible for yellow-fat disease, "a generalized disorder of fatty depots observed in a wide variety of animals." Neither of these concerns has been substantiated by subsequent research, though a legitimate, ongoing concern is that omega-3s are more vulnerable than other fatty acids to attack by oxygen, producing highly reactive free radicals that in turn attack other molecules and tissues.

In the meantime, Dyerberg and Bang had returned to Greenland (without Sinclair) to find out if the high eicosapentaenoic content of the Eskimos' diet really does affect the time it takes for their blood to clot. Aase Nielsen, the technician on their first expedition, had observed a difference in bleeding time in 1970, and Bang and Dyerberg had read accounts of historic battles in which blood was described as flowing profusely from the wounds of Eskimos, as well as accounts of explorers who mentioned the Eskimos' propensity for nosebleeds.

"An extremely frequent disorder—if it is proper to use this name for a condition which the people mostly disregard—is the frequent nose bleedings," wrote the Arctic explorer Peter Freuchen, who correctly and presciently attributed this phenomenon to diet. "There is scarcely one individual of the tribe whose nose will not bleed spontaneously at least every fourth or fifth day." But Bang and Dyerberg were the first to actually measure the bleeding time of the Eskimos. They returned to their uncomplaining Eskimo subjects in the settlement of Igdlorssuit and were amazed when they found that the time it took for their blood to clot was almost twice that of Danish controls (8.1 minutes versus 4.8). The two Danish doctors returned home ecstatic. They thought they had solved the paradox of the Eskimos' low rate of heart disease and would save the world from this devastating and expensive illness.

(Back in England, the elderly Sinclair made headlines, but did nothing to increase his standing with the scientific community, by going on a diet of seal meat for one hundred days in order to observe the change in his own bleeding time. The seal was sent to him frozen from Canada, and the smell of it thawing and cooking in the dining rooms of Magdalen College at Oxford, where Sinclair took most of his evening meals, was enough to keep many of the other fellows away. Sinclair's bleeding time did increase, but no one could be sure that he hadn't acquired scurvy from this unbalanced diet. "The Eskimos eat every part of their animals—brains, bones, innards and meat," says Dyerberg, who has tried to distance himself from Sinclair's very unscientific scheme. "Sinclair was just eating the meat.")

Only later, with further research, did it become clear that Bang and Dyerberg had exposed only one aspect and one benefit of the Eskimo diet; in fact, the omega-3s in fish protect against heart disease in ways besides prolonging the bleeding time. They have a beneficial effect on blood pressure and on all the blood lipids, including serum cholesterol, as William Connor at the Oregon Health and Science University in Portland began reporting in 1983. Eicosapentaenoic acid has also been found to have a profound dampening effect on the inflammatory response in tissues (a response now thought to initiate many of the processes of heart disease). And DHA, which Dyerberg and Bang initially thought to be of little importance, has since been found to stabilize heart cells. Increased amounts of DHA in the membranes of heart cells, as the Boston physician Alexander Leaf discovered in 1995, greatly decrease the tendency of those cells to develop abnormal and potentially fatal rhythms, or arrhythmia, the most common immediate cause of death in persons with heart disease.

But even without knowledge of these additional effects, the results of Dyerberg and Bang's fourth trip to Greenland were compelling enough to inspire researchers to study the protective effects of eating fish and fish oil and to reexamine the data from Keys's Seven Countries Study. In England's Diet and Reinfarction Trial (DART), reported on in 1989, the protective effect of fish appeared within six months of the beginning of the study, a rapid response that was reminiscent of the rise and fall of heart disease during the Second World War. Researchers, however, were no longer mystified by sudden changes of this kind. They now understood the power of thromboxane and were beginning to understand the role of DHA in cell membranes.

Even more fundamentally, the results of Dyerberg and Bang's fourth trip to Greenland were changing scientists' views on what "normal" meant in terms of blood flow and many other very basic biological parameters. Up until the late 1970s, "normal" was what occurred in the dominant Western culture. Usually, it was assumed to be the American average. But Dyerberg and Bang showed that even such a fundamental thing as the time it took for blood to clot could be vastly different in different parts of the world and could be altered by such a simple means as diet.

"We must be very careful about the term 'normal'" says Dyerberg, "because 'normal' may be very far from optimal. Maybe the 'normal' bleeding time is closer to the Eskimos', and it is we who have the 'abnormal' shortened bleeding time. After all, what are we dying of? We're not dying of bleeding, are we? No, we're dying of clotting, which is a far more severe problem."

SIX

TREE LARD AND COW OIL

The mountain sheep are sweeter,
But the valley sheep are fatter;
We therefore deemed it meeter
To carry off the latter.

THOMAS LOVE PEACOCK, 1829

BEFORE I PICK UP THE TRAIL OF RALPH HOLMAN'S RESEARCH—FROM the 1960s, when he gave polyunsaturated fats their catchy names, to the 1970s and '80s, when he finally settled the matter of whether omega-3s were essential for humans—I'd like to spend some time on fat itself, that greasy substance that is the vehicle, or defining taste, of most cuisines. *Greasy* did not always have the derogatory connotation it does today. It used to be a compliment, but its meaning has changed as our diet has become sweeter. Together, fats and carbohydrates make up more than 80 percent of the calories in every diet consumed by humankind. As one goes up, the other goes down—in concentration, as well as popularity.

Fat has fallen out of favor as sugar consumption has increased and physicians (until, at least, the recent Atkins craze) have voiced concerns about its health effects, but it has never lost its flavor, if you will forgive the small play on words. Grease, fat, blubber, oil, lard, tallow, butter, suet—whatever name you give to this substance that is insoluble in water, it is the source of most of the flavors of foods. And that is because aroma molecules are also insoluble in water but very soluble in fats. So fat gives foods their distinctive aromas and tastes. It is the vehicle of what we think of as cuisine. Whale blubber is every bit as connected with the Eskimos' sense of how foods should smell and taste as olive oil is for Italians, lard is for Mexicans, and sesame oil is for the Chinese. Some say that people even begin to smell like the fat they use in cooking. When Europeans first took up residence in China in the 1800s, the Chinese, who rarely use animal fats, thought that these foreigners smelled like butter, or cow oil, as they sometimes called it.

Others can write more eloquently and mouthwateringly about the role of fats in cuisine than I. When I said I wanted to spend some time on fat, I meant the structure of fats, not the foods they flavor and define. This sounds like more chemistry, but don't worry. Most of us have a pretty good idea of the structure of fats, especially those we cook with.

We know, for example, that butter, coconut oil, and palm oil are solids at a room temperature of about 72 degrees Fahrenheit, which is the reason that palm oil is sometimes called tree lard. And it is just a short step to understanding that this solidity comes from the high percentage of saturated fatty acids (such as stearic and palmitic acid) in each of these fats. The regular, zigzagging tails of saturated fats, with little of the bending or flexibility that double bonds introduce, make it easy for them to stack neatly on one another, giving rise to crystals or solids.

Cooks know something about unsaturated fats, too, though they may not know that they know it. They know that certain fats are much more likely to go rancid and to develop off flavors if they are exposed to air. They know that beef keeps longer in the freezer than pork; pork, longer than fish. And, again, it is only a short step to learning that these differences arise from

Stearic acid: +69°C

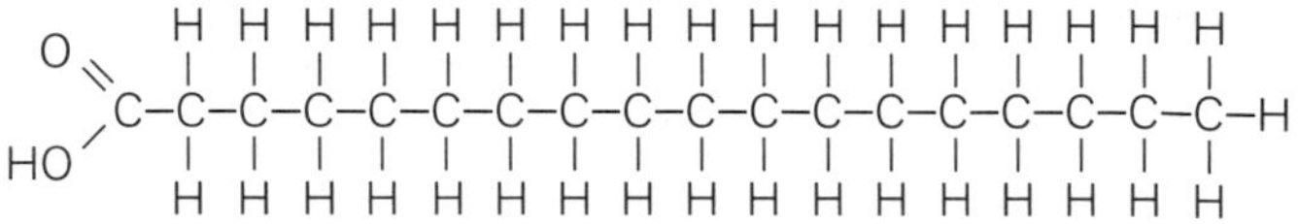

Oleic acid: +13°C

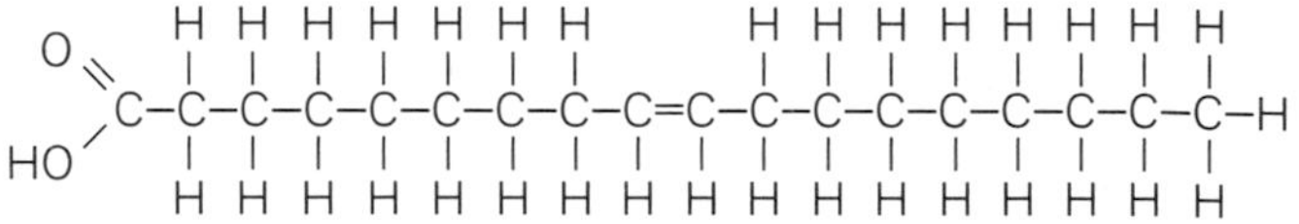

Linoleic acid: −9°C

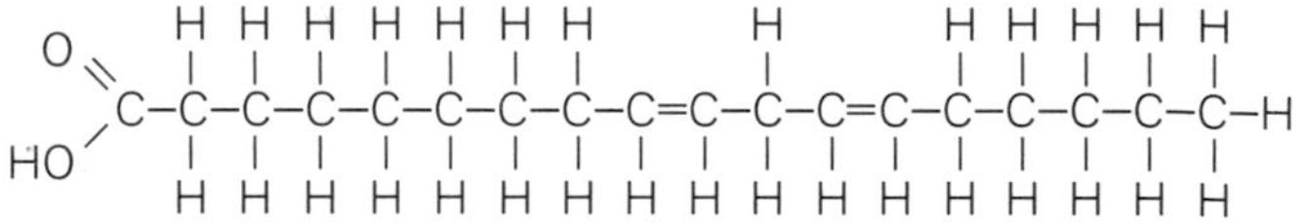

Alpha linolenic acid: −17°C

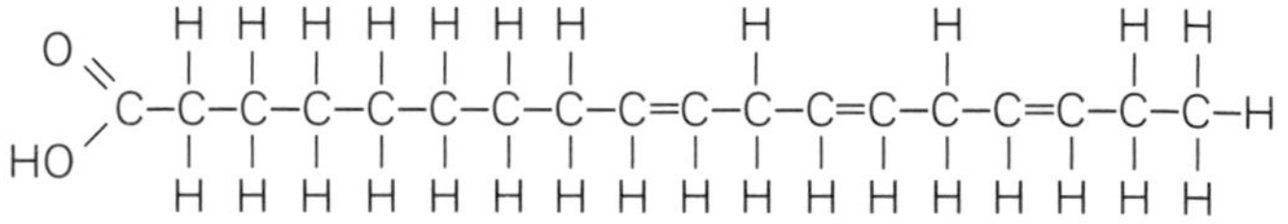

FIGURE 5 The melting point, the temperature at which a solid becomes a liquid, tells us something about the role that double bonds play in fats—and in nature. All these fatty acids are eighteen carbons long, but only one, stearic acid, is a solid at room temperature. The rest, with one, two, and three double bonds, are liquids. Changing the usual cis configuration of a double bond also has a profound effect on the melting point; the trans form of oleic acid, for example, has a melting point of 44°C (111°F), up from 13°C (55°F). Melting points do not tell the whole story,

the increasing amounts of double bonds in the fats of each of these foods, because the hydrogen atoms on either side of a double bond are very vulnerable to attack by oxygen molecules. Oxidized fats are not a good thing—either in the kitchen or in living tissues. Plants and animals protect their fats against attack with antioxidants, kamikaze-like molecules that are designed to take the oxygen hit and leave the fat intact. Cooks protect against oxidation by serving foods when they are fresh, by covering foods with plastic wrap, and by using refrigeration. Short of that, they serve foods made with hydrogenated or partially hydrogenated vegetable oils, oils in which the number of double bonds has been reduced.

Cooks also know that fat is the most energy-dense food, providing more than twice the amount of calories as carbohydrates or proteins (9 calories per gram versus 4). They understand that they must use enough fat in their cooking so that their meals will be filling and satisfying but not so much that their guests won't be tempted to try the dessert they've made. The increased energy in fats comes from the dense packing of their carbon-to-carbon and carbon-to-hydrogen bonds, all of which can be bro-

---

though, since DHA has a slightly higher melting point than some fatty acids with fewer double bonds. Also important to the behavior of fatty acids is the sequencing of their double bonds and whether any of their carbons lie between two double bonds. The hydrogens on this type of conjugated carbon, as it is called, are extremely reactive—with oxygen and enzymes. And they make it easier for the molecule to rapidly change shape. Alpha linolenic acid has four of these hydrogens, arachidonic acid has six, and DHA has ten. Linoleic acid has two.

ken and the released energy used as fuel. Proteins have amine groups that can't be broken down and must be excreted in the urine; much of the space in carbohydrates is taken up by large oxygen atoms. The caloric content of fats or oils is said to be 120 calories per tablespoon, but unsaturated fats can have slightly less because a double bond contains about 10 percent less energy than a single bond. This difference might help explain why dieters are more successful when they include lots of fish in their diet plan—but there are other reasons as well, as a later chapter will discuss.

Plants and animals store their excess energy as both fat and carbohydrates, but plants store much more energy as carbohydrates and animals store much more energy as fat. The space-saving, energy-dense qualities of fat are important to plants when they are producing seeds, but they are important to animals, which must move around in order to find food and mates, at all times. If the fat supply of a 120-pound woman were converted to carbohydrates, she would weigh about 150 pounds and would have lost much of her agility and swiftness. There is no limit to the amount of fat that humans can store, a great advantage in times of unpredictable food supplies and a considerable drawback, at times like now, when food is always abundant.

Cooks also know something else important about fat: fat and water, oil and water don't mix. This is a problem for cooks when they are making salad dressings or gravies. It is a problem for all living things since tissues are mostly water and fat must be prevented from gumming up these delicate works. Animals address the difficulty by attaching fats to a polar group, which *is* water soluble, and by packaging and repackaging fat every time it is moved anywhere in the body in proteins that have both a hydrophobic and hydrophilic side. Cooks use an emulsifier like lecithin.

Lecithin is a naturally occurring substance found in egg yolks and is the culinary equivalent of soap, says Harold McGee, who writes about the science of everyday life. It bridges the gap between fats and water and is, in fact, a kind of phospholipid, a compound I described in chapter 1 as the building block of membranes.

All phospholipids look like triglycerides in which one of the hydrocarbon tails has been replaced by a strongly polar phosphate group—a seemingly small change, but one that enables these molecules to do amazing things. In living tissues, they create one of the wonders of the biological world, the bilayers of membranes: self-assembling, multilayered structures (a kind of lipid sandwich) in which the negative phosphate groups (the bread) line up on the outside, in contact with the watery environment on the inside and outside of cells, and the fatty tails (the peanut butter) tuck themselves in the middle. There they form a barrier to water and other charged molecules.

This all goes to show that the natural antipathy between water and fat isn't just a problem for animals and plants, something they put up with in order to take advantage of the extra calories in fat. It's also something they put to work for them. Living things use this chemical aversion between lipids and water (this hostility, as Herman Melville calls it in *Moby-Dick*) to build the thin, water-resistant barriers that separate cells from cells and cells into parts, the membranes that make multicellular life possible.

I could go on and on about the things cooks know about fats, but there are certain things that cooks can't know about fats unless their kitchen is also a laboratory. One of these is the great diversity of fatty acids that make up any of the fats we know, such as butter or corn oil. Cooks take advantage of this multiformity when they serve ice cream or when they place a pat of butter on

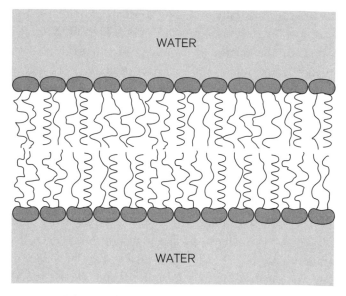

FIGURE 6 Bilayers of phospholipids form the backbone of every cell membrane. The hydrophilic parts of these phospholipids (the polar phosphate groups) are exposed to water; the hydrophobic parts (the fatty tails) are shielded from it.

a scoop of mashed potatoes to slowly melt, which it wouldn't do if the triglycerides in the butter didn't contain numerous different fatty acids, all with different melting points.

But this diversity is hard to recognize, especially in something that looks as homogeneous as a stick of butter or a hunk of lard. What cook would suspect, as chemists first began showing in the 1950s and '60s, that there are dozens of different fatty acids, making up hundreds of different triglycerides, in most fats? In part this diversity functions to prevent the formation of crystals, sharp things that could punch holes in cells, and in part it helps cells to create just the right environment in their membranes for proteins to twist and turn. What that environment is and how animals maintain it, how it is affected by diet and fine-tuned for different organs, are still largely mysteries—to biologists as well as cooks. But they are mysteries, remember, of which Keys and other lipid hypothesizers were hardly even aware.

SEVEN

THE CHEMIST IN THE KITCHEN

Thy food shall be thy remedy.

ATTRIBUTED TO HIPPOCRATES, CA. 400 B.C.E.

NO ONE KNOWS MORE ABOUT THE DIVERSITY OF FATTY ACIDS IN FAT than Ralph Holman. He spent years, decades, teasing out alpha linolenic acid (or eicosapentaenoic acid or DHA) from the messy mixture of triglycerides that make up any one fat. In the process, he acquired an appreciation for those messy mixtures. There must be some reason for them, though neither scientist nor cook understood it as yet.

This appreciation kept him from jumping on the prostaglandin bandwagon as so many scientists did in the 1960s and '70s. Holman heard through the grapevine about his good friend Sune Bergström's success in isolating these powerful new biological messengers. And when Bergström and David van Dorp published their papers in 1964, he learned, along with the rest of the scientific world, that fatty acids were the starting material of prostaglandins.

But Holman did not think, as many did, that the role of essential fatty acids was now completely understood and that it was only to provide the starting material of prostaglandins. With his intimate knowledge of the behavior of different fats, he suspected that polyunsaturates play other important roles in the body: in transporting cholesterol, as he had been suggesting since the 1950s, and in creating the optimal environment of membranes, which are involved in most metabolic processes.

"While Bergström would be looking for ways to increase his yield of prostaglandins," Holman told me in a recent telephone conversation, "I'd be looking for ways to prevent fatty acids from turning into prostaglandins. Bergström was only interested in prostaglandins and threw everything else away. I was interested in everything that came before the prostaglandins."

Ever since his collaboration with the pediatrician Arild Hansen on the problem of eczema in bottle-fed infants (changing the once-common practice of feeding babies sweetened skim milk), Holman had been intrigued by the connection between essential fatty acids and disease. At first, this meant examining only linoleic acid and arachidonic acid, since those were the only fats that could correct the symptoms seen by the Burrs. And at first, the only animals shown to have an absolute requirement for these fats were rats; then, because of his work with Hansen, human infants.

The essentialness of linoleic acid for adults was an unresolved question, as I noted in chapter 3, until the 1960s, when hospitals became capable of maintaining patients on intravenous feeding, or total parenteral nutrition (TPN), for longer and longer periods of time. Because of the difficulties of delivering lipids intravenously (fat being insoluble in an aqueous solution), the first TPN preparations were fat-free. Patients who were sustained on them for long periods developed many of the same symptoms that the Burrs' rats had displayed thirty years before: dry scaly skin, weight loss, and an increase in water consumption.

Tragically, Ralph Holman's mother was one of these patients. She was put on TPN after a mesenteric infarction destroyed the use of her bowels, and Holman watched helplessly as she died of the very kind of deficiency that he was working to prevent. His mother's doctor was receptive to what Holman was telling him about essential fatty acids (as many doctors at the time were not), but neither of them could figure out how to safely provide her with the nutrients she was missing. Unmodified fat given intravenously could itself cause death. Rubbing her body with corn oil, which they tried, was somewhat effective but couldn't entirely correct the deficiency. A nontoxic fat emulsion was developed in Sweden in 1961, but it was not yet available in the United States. In 1962, Holman's mother died.

"Why would this happen to my mother of all people?" Holman remembers asking himself, and he redoubled his efforts to convince the medical profession of the importance of fats. Not knowing what he would find, he asked physicians who specialized in diseases of the nervous system for blood samples from their patients. That was when he got his first hint that a deficiency of omega-3 fats was a much more widespread problem in human health than a lack of omega-6s.

By that time it was known that brains and nerves are very rich in the long-chain polyunsaturated fatty acids—arachidonic acid, as well as DHA. Holman had a hunch that patients with anorexia nervosa, Huntington's disease, macular degeneration, multiple sclerosis, neuronal degeneration, retinitis pigmentosa, and Reye's syndrome would be deficient in arachidonic acid. To his great surprise, these patients usually had plenty of arachidonic acid, but they had very small amounts of the omega-3 fatty acid DHA.

Holman was a member of the American Oil Chemists Society and began presenting these findings at its meetings. The reaction was "So what? What makes you think that these low levels of DHA are the cause, and not the result, of these diseases?" Undiscouraged by this response, Holman decided that he needed to get an idea of the fatty acids in healthy people. So he began collecting blood samples from populations around the world. He would compare them to a group from Minnesota.

He expected that his Minnesota controls, one hundred citizens from the richest country in the world, would come out well compared to, say, people in India. But he was amazed to find that this group was at the bottom of the scale in terms of the amount of omega-3 fatty acids in their tissues and near the top of the scale in terms of the amount of omega-6 fatty acids. The only populations Holman looked at that ranked lower than these Minnesota controls in their levels of omega-3 fatty acids (including populations from Sweden and Australia, as well as India and, later, Nigeria) were a group of malnourished Argentine infants and a group of American infants.

But these data, too, were little more than a curiosity at first, inspiring little response beyond "So what?" Omega-3 fatty acids had never been shown to be essential for humans, so why should it matter that their content in blood cells was less than 4 percent in American infants and more than 13 percent in Nigerians, or that DHA levels were so low in American populations? Such results just showed that a broad range of these fatty acids could sustain life.

In 1967, omega-3 fatty acids had been found to be essential for trout (when it was observed that trout on a corn oil diet didn't grow as well and had a much higher death rate than trout on a fish diet), but it was thought that the requirements of fish differ from those of mammals. "The well-known differences in the composition of marine and mammalian body lipids support the supposition of differing fatty acid requirements," the authors of this study wrote. "The fatty acids of fish are more unsaturated . . . and fatty acids of the linolenic type predominate." This made sense to investigators, since cold aquatic environments demand higher degrees of unsaturation than terrestrial environ-ments. Few thought the requirement for omega-3s might be widespread.

Then, in the late 1970s, a number of developments cast Hol-man's research in a new light and began suggesting that the king of fats, linoleic acid, had a queen. Dyerberg and Bang's work with the Eskimos showed that there were important health conse-quences to different tissue concentrations of eicosapentaenoic acid. And Holman was asked to consult in the case of a gunshot victim, a six-year-old girl, who had been accidentally shot in the stomach by her caretaker's husband.

Shawna Renee Strobel was a blond, blue-eyed, healthy kin-dergartner at the time she suffered the wound that would make her the first human case of omega-3 deficiency ever to be re-corded in the scientific literature. Her mother, Dorena Strobel, worked as a waitress in a family-style restaurant in the small town of Morris, Illinois, on the Illinois River. Another young waitress, Doris Clark, who was married but unable to have children, became attached to both Dorena and her young daughter. She volunteered to babysit Shawna when Dorena was working, and she invited Shawna to spend the night on several occasions, including Halloween of October 1978, when she and her hus-band wanted to take the six-year-old to the town's festivities.

Doris picked Shawna up from her house on the afternoon of Halloween, and Shawna's mother didn't see her daughter again until she was being lifted from the floor of the Clarks' car in front of the small hospital in Morris. "He told me to tell you it was an accident but it wasn't," Dorena remembers Shawna saying before she passed out. Ray Clark, Doris's husband, did indeed tell the police that Shawna had shot herself in the stomach. Later, it was determined that his .22-caliber rifle had gone off while he was cleaning it in the living room. Clark spent six months in a correctional facility.

Shawna, meanwhile, was undergoing numerous operations to save her life and what remained of her intestines. In the first seven days after the accident, she had three surgeries that removed eight feet of her small intestine and one foot of her large intestine, as well as her ileocecal valve. Later, at the Children's Memorial Hospital in Chicago, surgeons would reconnect her remaining intestines with protoplastic, which would spare her, if she survived, the necessity of wearing a colostomy bag to collect her stools. But the removal of so much intestine and colon ensured that all of Shawna's nutrition would have to come from TPN. Total parenteral nutrition was much improved since the time when Holman's mother died—it now included linoleic acid. But it was still far from perfect, as this six-year-old would show.

After a half a year of operations and recuperation, Shawna was discharged to her mother's care at home, and Dorena, who says she had always wanted to be a nurse, learned nursing the hard way. She learned how to hook her daughter up to the medical infusion pump and how to sterilize all her feeding tubes. Shawna was doing as well as could be expected, her doctors thought, until November of the following year. Then she began having episodes of tingling, numbing, and weakness in her legs, sometimes accompanied by blurred vision and a total inability to walk. It was a peculiar array of symptoms that the neurologists treating her had never seen before.

Given all that Shawna had been through, some of her physicians thought her problems were more psychological than physical. But one, Terry Hatch, at the Carle Foundation Hospital at the University of Illinois, suspected that her intravenous nutrition was somehow responsible and contacted a nutrition researcher.

This researcher had done part of his training at the University of Minnesota and happened to know of Holman's research. So Holman was asked to do a fatty acid analysis of the lipids in Shawna's blood.

Holman never met Shawna or her mother, but he saved the Illinois girl's life when he determined that the amount of omega-3 fatty acids in the girl's serum was about one-third that of controls. Holman also looked at the TPN preparation that the girl was on, which was based on safflower oil, and found that it, too, was very low in omega-3 fatty acids. At the time, safflower oil had the reputation of being a very healthy oil because of its high polyunsaturate (and low saturate) content. But its ratio of omega-6 fatty acids to omega-3 fatty acids is about 115 to 1. That ratio, as Holman knew from his experiments exploring metabolic competition, would prevent many omega-3 fats from getting into Shawna's tissues. Picture 115 women and 1 man all trying to get through the same small door. Though the man is bigger and can push through the crowd, he doesn't stand much of a chance.

Holman suggested that Shawna be put on a different TPN preparation, one based on soybean oil and containing both linoleic and alpha linolenic acids (in a ratio of 6 to 1). In twelve weeks, all of her neurological symptoms had disappeared. She lived until the age of twenty-two, when she died of a stroke after a small bowel transplant. It was a short life, but much longer than anyone had expected and longer than would have been possible without Holman's intervention. Shawna had graduated from college and was living on her own at the time she died. She was only vaguely aware that she had made medical history.

Holman and Hatch published their findings about the young gunshot victim in the *American Journal of Clinical Nutrition* in 1982, the same year that Holman was elected to the National Academy of Sciences, but the reaction was, again, "So what?"

What does it matter if alpha linolenic acid is essential for humans, when it is almost impossible to make someone deficient in this fat? Human bodies require very little of it in their diets (about 0.5 percent of their calories), and it is everywhere in the food supply—except the very limited food supply of Shawna Strobel.

Another reaction was "What's new?" George and Mildred Burr discussed linolenic acid as a possible essential fatty acid in 1930; thus Holman just proved what had been suspected all along. It didn't seem to matter to these skeptics that Shawna's symptoms were very different from those of the Burrs' rats: dizziness and blurred vision versus scaly skin. They didn't seem to grasp that this was an entirely new deficiency. "I don't think the case made a lot of impact," says Hatch. "The solution was at hand—a new formula—so the problem didn't seem all that important." It was a piece in a puzzle that wasn't yet known to exist.

But for Holman and a few other researchers, Shawna's case brought a sea change in attitudes, a new way of looking at the world. Shawna told Holman that it was possible to become deficient in omega-3 fatty acids. And if that was true, then maybe we ought to be paying attention to where these fats are in the food supply and how they survive food-processing techniques. Maybe eicosapentaenoic acid, the fat that Dyerberg and Bang had brought to the world's attention, should be thought of not as an important supplement that could *prevent* heart disease but as a nutrient whose absence was helping to *cause* heart disease.

Holman put this information together and began proselytizing to family and friends. When one of the employees at the Hormel Institute was suffering from heart failure and was at home on disability leave, Holman would stop by with cookies and cakes he had made with flaxseed and flaxseed oil. "If I were you," he told Dale Jarvis, "I would be taking fish oil." Holman stopped by so often that Jarvis, who already had undergone one bypass operation and had been told by his doctors that he had no functioning arteries that could be repaired, finally asked his physician for permission to try fish oil. He became one of the first people to take massive doses of fish oil to correct a heart problem, a treatment now widely recommended. This was in 1985, when today's ubiquitous fish oil capsules were nowhere to be found, so Holman bought it in bulk, in large cans, and began working Jarvis up to 12 grams (about a tablespoon) a day. It was pretty awful, since fish oil has a "bad aftertaste and it was hard to take that much of it," recalls Jarvis, but he kept at it because the improvement in his angina was almost immediate.

Within a few days, Jarvis was up and pushing his lawn mower. Within a few weeks, he was back at his job at the institute, taking care of its instruments; one of his first projects was to build a device to put fish oil into capsules. Later that year, he went on vacation to the Grand Tetons and rode horseback at 12,000 feet. Meanwhile, Holman was taking blood samples from Jarvis to see how the structural lipids, the phospholipids, in the membranes of his red blood cells were changing. All his omega-3s were low at first, but his eicosapentaenoic acid level was particularly low— less than half that of Minnesota controls. It soon jumped to four times that of the controls.

"My wife thinks the sun rises and sets on Ralph Holman," says Jarvis, who had more than two decades of good health before he had a second coronary bypass operation. "My doctors didn't have any advice for me, other than rest, but they thought that the fish oil wouldn't hurt. After two months, they said, 'Whatever you're doing, it's working.'"

Jarvis could tolerate the fish oil, but for some reason, he couldn't tolerate the flaxseed cakes that Holman used to bring him. With that caveat, I include the recipe for Holman's cake I found in his unpublished memoir. It is for readers to try, or just to read for the insights it offers into Holman. Like all good recipes, this one says as much about the cook as the dish—and the cook, in this case, is a big-hearted chemist who was always generous with his knowledge and his food.

RALPH'S OMEGA-3 POLYUNSATURATED CAKE

Equipment: 7" round bottom bowl; rubber spatula;
Teflon-lined baking pan, 7 1/2" × 12"

To bowl add:
  2 eggs (without shells)
  1/8 cup canola oil
  1 1/2 cups 2 percent milk
  2 teaspoons sodium free baking powder
  4 teaspoons almond flavoring (or butter flavoring, if
      you are in a dairy state of mind)
  1/2 cup milled flax
  1 cup sugar
  3/4 cup chopped walnuts
  2 cups whole wheat graham flour

Mix thoroughly with spatula.
Bake at 325 degrees F.

Don't worry about the cholesterol in the eggs. If you get your omega-3 acids, they will take care of the cholesterol.

Omega-3s are the principal PUFAs [polyunsaturated fatty acids] of brain and nerve. You are seeing these words and thinking with omega-3 acids right now.

This recipe contains canola oil, flaxmeal, and walnuts, all of which are rich sources of alpha linolenic acid, $18:3\omega3$.

You may eat this cake with a clear conscience.

EIGHT

OUT OF AFRICA . . .

The best food is that which fills the belly.

ARABIC PROVERB

IN THIS BRIEF TELLING OF THE LONG HISTORY OF HOW SCIENTISTS discovered the importance of omega-3 fatty acids, I've had to reduce the cast of characters enormously, as the reader has probably surmised. Out of the complicated tapestry of people and ideas that make up any new field of science, I've focused on the most dominant colors or threads. And in the process, I know, I've slighted some great scientists and great science. I've barely mentioned the work of the innovative fish biologist Robert Ackman, and I've said nothing yet about Howard Sprecher, the biochemist who worked out the complete pathway for the synthesis of DHA from alpha linolenic acid.

But there are two scientists, William Lands and Michael Crawford, who have been as significant in shaping this history as Ralph Holman, Jørn Dyerberg, and Hans Olaf Bang, and it is time I gave them their due. I'll begin with the English biochemist Crawford, who currently heads the Institute of Brain Chemistry and Human Nutrition at the London Metropolitan University, not because he's older than Lands (in fact he's younger, though they're both in their seventies) but because his ideas about fats and human nutrition were shaped in Africa, where we all began.

"Africa was an awakening," Crawford told me when I visited him in his office in north London in the fall of 2003. "The diseases of Western societies were almost nonexistent, but the people suffered from a wide panorama of very different diseases—many of which had an obvious connection to diet. They didn't have atherosclerosis, but their hearts failed from endomyocardial fibrosis, due to diets too low in protein. They didn't have diabetes or arthritis, but they did have liver cancer from consuming peanuts contaminated with aflatoxins."

Fresh out of graduate school in 1960, Crawford was made the head of the department of biochemistry at the Makerere University Medical School in Kampala, Uganda. He traveled extensively in Africa over the next five years, sometimes with his wife and two children. He was amazed at how sharply disease patterns could change over distances of just hundreds of miles.

On one particularly treacherous expedition to the shores of Lake Rudolph in northern Kenya, Crawford and a number of other researchers and physicians crossed many miles of lava desert to see if they could determine what was causing the bowed legs of a small tribe of people called the El Molo. The people had legs that looked like sabers or like the legs of children with severe rickets, a deficiency of vitamin D. The tribe was separated from other people by the barren landscape that surrounds Lake Rudolph, and all of its food and water came from the lake. But the lake water, these researchers found, was extremely alkaline; in addition, the diet of these people, mostly fish, was very low in calcium. For those reasons, not genetics or infection, the shins of the El Molo, their weight-bearing bones, were weak and bowed.

On another trip—to the very fertile shores of Lake Victoria, where a wealthy and sophisticated tribe of people called the

Bugandans lived off the large green bananas that grow like weeds there—Crawford was shocked to see tribesmen driving their malnourished children to the hospital in cars. The sale of these green bananas, or plantains, and coffee has helped the Bugandans grow wealthy but not healthy, since plantains are low in protein and what protein they do have is deficient in several amino acids.

Adults can survive on this food source if it is supplemented with small amounts of meat and vegetables, but children, with their fast growth rates and smaller stomachs, are prone to malnutrition. Their growth is often arrested, and they develop the potbelly that is characteristic of protein calorie malnutrition, or kwashiorkor. The plantain diet can cause problems even for adults, who may regularly eat more than two pounds of plantains at a sitting. That amount of food can cause intestinal obstructions—painful and potentially fatal twists in the gut that are the Bugandans' major reason for surgery.

These experiences and others convinced Crawford that "food really matters." The popularity of Keys's lipid hypothesis in the 1960s led him to develop the theory (which he now knows is oversimplified) that protein consumption, or underconsumption, is the major problem in Africa and that fat consumption, or overconsumption, is the major problem in the West. So when Crawford returned to London in 1965 to set up a new laboratory at the Nuffield Institute of Comparative Medicine, he decided to focus on lipid research. He outfitted his lab with a new gas-liquid chromatograph (courtesy of Jack Heinz, chairman of the American food company, who had both a personal and a professional interest in nutrition) and obtained standards for eicosapentaenoic acid, DHA, and arachidonic acid from the Hormel Institute in Minnesota.

Crawford saw no reason to approach lipid research from the point of view of the heart and the vascular system, an already overcrowded field. However, there was an organ that was mostly fat—60 percent fat—which few were studying: the brain.

In Africa, Crawford had eaten a great deal of wild game and had been intrigued by the relationship of an animal's brain to its carcass. He had observed large animals, like the wildebeest and eland, with small brains, as well as small animals, like the jackal, with relatively large brains and had wondered about the reason for this mismatch in brain and body size. Back in England, he took a roundabout approach to this question by first studying the fat composition of the bodies of wild African animals, animals he obtained from the Uganda Game Department. Crawford compared the fat of these wild animals to that of domesticated animals and of cod liver oil, which he got from Robert Ackman in Nova Scotia. He learned that the fats in the tissues of wild animals were much less saturated than the fats in the tissues of domesticated animals. It was the chemistry behind what anyone who has ever dealt with wild and domesticated flesh already knows: the fats of wild animals are softer and less solid than those of domesticated animals.

At the time of these early experiments, animal fat was frequently spoken of as the villain in heart disease. But Crawford realized that the fats of animals change dramatically with diet, a point he made in a very controversial 1968 article in the *New Scientist*, "Are Our Cows Killing Us?" The total fat content of the domestic cow was considerably greater than its wild counterpart, Crawford reported in this piece (which seems even better suited to the year 2005 than to 1968), and the polyunsaturate content was much smaller, 2 percent versus the approximately 30 percent in free-living animals.

In 1968, Crawford was also put in charge of organizing a symposium for the Zoological Society of London, and he invited Hugh Sinclair to speak on nutrition and atherosclerosis. Like

Dyerberg and Bang, he was unaware of Sinclair's reputation as a dilettante, but he had read Sinclair's piece in the *Lancet* and was impressed by his idea that heart disease resulted from a chronic deficiency of essential fatty acids in the diet. (By essential fatty acids, remember, Sinclair meant the fats of both the omega-6 and omega-3 families.)

Crawford adopted this idea as he continued his comparisons of animal fats; but as soon as he began looking at the fats that make up the brains of different mammals, he shifted his attention to the omega-3 fats. For when he turned from bodies to brains, he found something very unusual. While the fats in most tissues and organs vary with the species—and its diet—and the specific organ, the fats of brains did not. No matter which of the forty-four species of mammals Crawford looked at (and he looked at everything from fruit-eating bats to leopards), no matter what it ate or the size of its brain, a little over a tenth of the fats in that organ were arachidonic acid, an omega-6 fat that is common throughout the body, and about a quarter were DHA, an omega-3 fat that is found in highest concentrations in brains and nervous tissue. Eicosapentaenoic acid was also present in brains but at extremely low levels.

Crawford's explanation for this remarkable finding is that DHA must be "rate limiting" in brain development, meaning that an animal's ability to consume or make DHA constrains the size of its brain. In time, he would develop this explanation into a theory and a book, in which he would also propose that humans evolved on the shores and coast of Africa, where DHA-rich fish would have been readily available, not the savannas, as is generally accepted.

Regardless of the validity of his evolutionary theory (which seems unlikely to me for several reasons, including archaeological evidence placing human origins on the savanna and the fact that DHA is made from alpha linolenic acid, the most abundant fat on the earth), Crawford's work had the unquestionable benefit of turning scientific attention to the presence of DHA in the brain and to the brain's evident preference for this very long, highly unsaturated fatty acid. Robert Anderson, a biochemist at the Baylor College of Medicine, had already identified DHA as a critical part of the mammalian eye when he found that DHA was packed in the membranes of rod cells. Crawford's work established a larger context for this finding: the context of all brains and nervous tissue.

At first, researchers assumed that DHA was important to brains because it was converted into biologically active compounds, much as the twenty-carbon arachidonic and eicosapentaenoic acids were converted into prostaglandins. A great deal of time and effort were expended looking for the metabolites of DHA, and though several were found, none had anything like the potency of prostaglandins. Researchers eventually concluded that DHA does not exert its effects through metabolites and is concentrated in the brain and excitable tissues for other reasons. Those reasons have to do with the way it behaves in cell membranes.

Thus the omega-3 research was divided into two story lines: the prostaglandin story, dominated by arachidonic and eicosapentaenoic acid, and the membrane story, dominated by DHA. Many of the most powerful prostaglandins have been known since the 1970s (though new prostaglandins, now called eicosanoids, are discovered every year), but DHA has only recently begun to give up its secrets. For now, suffice it to say that its powerful and subtle effects in membranes (all membranes, but especially the membranes of excitable cells) go far beyond oxidation rates and melting points, far beyond what cooks can learn about fats in their kitchens.

Crawford, meanwhile, was continuing to compare the fats in different species—in herbivores and carnivores, for instance, and in different types of herbivores—when an event in his personal life took him into the unexpected arena of infant nutrition. He and his wife adopted a three-month-old infant (their third child), and Crawford wanted to make sure that whatever formula they chose would provide this baby with all the necessary nutrients. He was particularly concerned about fats, which make up more than half the available energy in formulas and human milk. He therefore used his gas-liquid chromatograph to analyze the infant formulas that were currently available in England. What he found was that all were lacking the most highly unsaturated fatty acids— eicosapentaenoic acid, arachidonic acid, and DHA—fats that were, as Crawford discovered by this same means, present in human breast milk. Interestingly, these fats were present in much greater amounts in the breast milk of women than in their blood cells, suggesting that they are somehow concentrated in milk to enhance the baby's development after birth.

In retrospect, the absence of these fats from formulas of the 1970s is not at all surprising, since these formulas were made with seed oils and most plants are unable to produce the longer and more unsaturated fatty acids.* But it was very disturbing to Crawford, given his understanding of brains and their high concentrations of DHA and arachidonic acid. Also disturbing were the high levels of linoleic acid in the formulas that Crawford tested—and the negligible levels of alpha linolenic acid. If babies were able to elongate and desaturate these parent fatty acids with

---

*It is thought that plants lost the ability to produce the longer and more desaturated fatty acids as they moved onto dry land. There, they would have benefited from a loss of flexibility and a firmer structure when it came to forming their stems, stalks, and trunks.

great efficiency (as they cannot), they might have enough arachidonic acid, but they would still be deficient in DHA.

Very few parents, pediatricians, or researchers would have recognized this deficiency as a problem, since neither alpha linolenic acid nor DHA had yet been recognized as being essential for babies, or humans of any age. But Crawford began supplementing his adopted child's formula with brains purchased from his butcher. He knew that brains were a traditional weaning food and "these were the days before mad cow disease," he explains.

Crawford also began to investigate what would happen to animals that were deficient in DHA by raising young capuchin monkeys on a diet in which the only fat was corn oil. Corn oil, with a ratio of linoleic acid to alpha linolenic acid of about 50 to 1, was, at the time, touted as the healthiest of all oils and was the basis of many infant formulas. But Crawford's monkeys developed skin lesions and patchy coats on their corn oil diets, and two of the eight monkeys developed a persistent self-mutilating behavior, gnawing at their genitalia and stomachs, and eventually had to be destroyed.

Upon autopsy, Crawford found far fewer omega-3 fatty acids in the tissues of these monkeys than in the tissues of monkeys who were fed linseed oil. "Whilst the possibility of a linolenic acid requirement for capuchins needs further investigation with a larger number of animals," Crawford and his colleagues cautiously concluded, "it is nevertheless difficult at the moment to find any interpretation for the results, other than linolenic acid deficiency."

At the same time, Crawford embarked on what would be a very long campaign to change infant formulas, a campaign that would pit him against powerful food interests. Alpha linolenic acid is the most abundant fat on earth, as I've said, but it is much less abundant in most seeds and seed oils than linoleic acid, which makes it more expensive than the latter. Also, alpha linolenic acid is much more prone to oxidation and much more likely to develop rancid and off flavors than its omega-6 cousin, making it a food manufacturer's nightmare. Plants and other living creatures protect against oxidation with antioxidants such as vitamin C and E, but these, too, are expensive additions to any food product. Science hadn't recognized the omega-3 fatty acids as being essential to humans, the formula companies pointed out; so why should they take on these additional costs and problems?

No one was ready to listen to Crawford in the early 1970s, when he first realized that infant formulas differed markedly from human milk in their fat content. He was disappointed, though, when there was a similar lack of attention to a report by the World Health Organization in 1977, which concluded that "the ideal recommendation for milk substitutes would be to match the essential fatty acids of human milk from well-nourished mothers with respect to both parent and long-chain essential fatty acids and the balance of n-6 to n-3 families of fatty acids." (This balance was reported to be about 5 to 1 though it, too, varies with diet. It is higher in the milk of American mothers and lower in the milk of the fish-eating Japanese and Eskimo mothers.)

"We all thought that having a report that came out of the best international scientific brains, going through the most rigorous processes, would change the situation for those infants that weren't receiving these nutrients through breast milk," Crawford remembers, "but the formula companies fought hard to maintain the status quo. They thought that they had already done babies a service by taking cow's milk out of their formulas and replacing it with vegetable oil—formulas they called 'humanized' because they contained linoleic acid."

In the 1980s, companies gradually began putting more alpha linolenic acid into their products. In the late '80s, Milupa in

Hamburg, Germany, became the first infant formula company to supplement its product with DHA and arachidonic acid. It had become clear that babies do have the enzymes to elongate and desaturate the parent fatty acids but that these reactions are so slow that unsupplemented babies will always have much less arachidonic acid and DHA than their breast-fed counterparts.

It wasn't until 2002, though, after supplemented formulas had become available in almost every other country in the world, that one went on sale in the United States. By then, there was a great deal of evidence, generated in laboratories in both the United States and England, that DHA could make a significant difference in an infant's visual acuity and mental development, including a 7-point difference on the Mental Development Index and a one-line difference on eye chart tests in infants one year of age.

Supplemented formulas are still just an option in this country. Parents must be educated enough to ask for them and wealthy enough to afford them. In one New York State grocery store in late 2004, one quart of Similac with DHA and arachidonic acid cost a dollar more, $5.99, than its unsupplemented counterpart; 12.9 ounces of Nestlé formula was $11.99 with supplements and $5.99 without. But they are an option that didn't exist three years ago, some thirty years after Crawford first discovered these important differences in breast milk and formula. No one knows how much brain power and visual acuity was lost in all the foot-dragging on the part of formula companies, but Crawford himself never missed an opportunity to press for change. He flew to the United States to testify before the Food and Drug Administration. He stood up in conference after conference in the 1980s and '90s, as numerous people have told me, and argued, "It's no longer up to the scientific community to justify why DHA should be in infant formula. It's up to the infant formula company to justify why it isn't."

NINE

... AND INTO THE MEMBRANE

Eat enough and it will make you wise.

JOHN LYLY, 1589

LIKE MICHAEL CRAWFORD, WILLIAM LANDS WAS ADVOCATING FOR dietary changes long before most scientists knew what an omega-3 fatty acid was and long before 1985, when a conference in Washington, D.C., left all the participants with the realization that there was something very wrong with the food supply. Lands arrived at this position not from his knowledge of brains, as Crawford had, but from his understanding of membranes, the very thin envelopes that surround every cell and every organelle within each cell, and of phospholipids, their basic building blocks.

Phospholipids, as Lands knew in the 1950s when he was beginning his research career, create the layers of these membranes spontaneously. They have polar heads, negatively charged phosphate groups, that group themselves on the outside, in contact with the aqueous environment on both the outside and the inside of cells, and two fatty tails that bury themselves in the middle. There, they line up with all the other fatty tails to form a double layer of fats, a barrier to water and other charged molecules.

But this barrier is also the window through which a cell does most of its business with the world. Ions must be transported across it; enzymes must be able to move around in it, often very rapidly. A membrane is an extremely busy place, crowded with proteins that span it and maneuver in it. It can't be made, at least entirely, of saturated fats, which are solid at body temperature and thus would impede all of this activity. One of a phospholipid's two tails is *always* an unsaturated fatty acid, and the other is *usually* a saturated fat, a fifty-fifty ratio that seems to give most membranes just the right amount of flexibility or liquidity, the consistency of a light engine oil. (Many of the phospholipids in the brain and the eye have two unsaturated tails, making that lubricant even lighter.)

This much was known in the 1950s. But how, Lands wondered as a young researcher at the University of Michigan, was this ratio achieved? How were phospholipids put together, and how did enzymes "know" whether a fatty acid was saturated or unsaturated? Lands discovered the enzymes that assembled phospholipids in the early 1960s (the acyltransferases) and began studying their preferences. He found that the enzyme that attaches the unsaturated chain to the phosphate group greatly prefers a fatty acid with at least twenty carbons and three double bonds. But it couldn't care less from what family that highly unsaturated fatty acid (known now to those in the business of fats as HUFAs, an elite class of polyunsaturates or PUFAs) comes.

As long as the chain has at least twenty carbons and three double bonds, the enzyme is just as happy attaching one of the omega-3 HUFAs (DHA or eicosapentaenoic acid) as it is one of the omega-6 HUFAs (arachidonic acid or the immediate precursor of arachidonic acid: dihomo-gamma-linolenic acid). It's content even to attach an omega-9 HUFA, Mead's acid (the only HUFA the body can manufacture from scratch), if it finds one, but Mead's acid is made only when the body is deficient in essential fatty acids.

This preference, or lack thereof, makes the acyltransferases very different, Lands realized, from the enzymes that Ralph Holman was then researching: the desaturases and elongases, which definitely prefer an omega-3 fatty acid at each step of the way. It meant that the body exercises only a limited amount of control over the fats that wind up in its membranes. At the time, Lands didn't think about the nutritional implications of his observation (other than that it fit in well with the current dogma, the one dividing fats into the healthy, unsaturated variety and the unhealthy, saturated kind). His foray into the realm of nutrition came a little later, after he realized that a second set of enzymes behaved in the same way.

In 1965, when it was learned that prostaglandins are made from arachidonic acid (and the other twenty-carbon fatty acids), Lands had a very good idea where the body would get its supply of these fats. "They don't just float around," says Lands. "They're the fats that wind up in phospholipids." So Lands bet Bengt Samuelsson, who went on to share a Nobel Prize with his former teacher, Sune Bergström, and with John Vane, that if our bodies were to make very much of the newly discovered prostaglandins, the arachidonic acid would come from the phospholipids in membranes.

This bet led to a 1967 sabbatical in Stockholm and a quick verification of Lands's hunch, followed by his discovery of the phospholipases—the enzymes that release the fatty acids from the membranes before they can be turned into prostaglandins. Lands returned home at the end of the year and, as a courtesy, waited a year or two to see if the scientists at the Karolinska Institute would follow up on this work. When it became clear that they were not interested in how prostaglandins were made, just the products themselves, he resumed his study of those enzymes.

The kinetics and the co-factors of these reactions were "just waiting to be discovered," as Lands says. Through 1971 and 1972, he made a discovery every month, including the effectiveness of eicosapentaenoic acid in slowing down the inflammatory reactions caused by prostaglandins (much as it slows down the thrombotic reactions caused by thromboxanes, as Dyerberg, Bang, and Vane would later show). Lands hypothesized at first that eicosapentaenoic acid was an inhibitor of the reaction that turned arachidonic acid into a potent mediator of inflammation, a reaction we now know is catalyzed by the COX enzyme. He later determined that it was a substrate (i.e., used in the reaction) rather than an inhibitor (i.e., something blocking the reaction), but a substrate that slowed the reaction down by a factor of at least five, so that the inflammatory response was almost negligible.

Another discovery, and the one that caused "an irretrievable veering of his career toward preventive medicine," as he wrote in a recent review, was that his new enzymes, the phospholipases, were also indifferent as to the family of the fat they snipped out of the membrane. As long as the fat was twenty carbons long, it didn't matter if it was the highly inflammatory arachidonic acid, the somewhat less inflammatory dihomo-gamma-linolenic acid (another omega-6 fat), or the placid, mediative eicosapentaenoic acid. They would even excise the twenty-carbon omega-9 fatty acid, which bodies make when they are deficient in essential fats. "Like the acyltransferases, these enzymes are promiscuous rather than selective," says Lands today. "They behave like the men in the old Rodgers and Hammerstein song: 'When they can't handle the hand they're fond of, they handle the hand they're near.'"

This promiscuity told Lands something very important in the 1970s, when he was first describing the enzymes' libertine behavior: you can change the kind of prostaglandin signaling in your body by changing the kinds of fats that you eat. You can change the balance between the "explosive signals" that arachidonic acid produces and the "little nudgy signals" that eicosapentaenoic acid produces by simple dietary choices about the kind of oil you cook with and about what you order, fish or beef.

As Lands was probably the first to realize, such adjustments could, in turn, change your tendency to develop certain diseases. At first, Lands was thinking only about arthritis-type diseases, since the earliest prostaglandins identified by Sune Bergström play a role in inflammation. Then, with the discovery of thromboxane, in 1975, Lands recognized the potential of diet in preventing heart disease by changing the tendency of platelets to aggregate, the first step in blood clotting. He saw that diet could reduce the necessity of taking aspirin, whose sole effect, as John Vane found, is to knock out the enzyme that makes these twenty-carbon messengers (the cyclooxygenase, or COX, enzyme). Aspirin is the most effective medicine in the cardiologist's black bag of treatments (better even than today's statins). In men, it cuts mortality from heart disease by more than half. But it can produce many harmful side effects, including gastric ulcers and kidney disease, which a simple change in diet would not. These side effects stem from aspirin's lack of discrimination in its effect on prostaglandin synthesis, as it wipes out both targeted and untargeted prostaglandins.

Diet can have the same effects as aspirin and aspirin-like drugs without their costs and negative side effects, Lands has been telling the world since the 1970s. Why the world hasn't listened is a good question and may have as much to do with the complexity of the science that is behind Lands's advice as with resistance on the part of food and pharmaceutical industries.

In the 1970s, pharmaceutical companies showed a great deal of interest in controlling prostaglandin synthesis, and Lands was frequently asked to be a consultant. He invented new ways of screening compounds for their anti-inflammatory effects and determined how the different anti-inflammatory drugs (acetaminophen and ibuprofen, for instance) affect prostaglandin synthesis differently than aspirin does. He always told the companies that nutrition would regulate the availability of prostaglandins too. And their answer was always the same: There's no way to make money from nutrition. Lands said the same thing about nutrition to John Vane when he met this very famous pharmacologist on a trip to Vienna. "Yes," he remembers Vane replying, "but you can't patent that."

Food companies such as Procter and Gamble, Kraft, and Campbell Soup were also curious about Lands's work and invited him to give presentations. "But they didn't want to touch the idea that they might be selling foods that were harmful to people with a ten-foot pole," says Lands. "Bill, we sell foods that people ask for," Lands recalls one executive explaining. "We don't tell the people what to eat. If you convince the public that our food should have a different balance, we'll change it."

So Lands has spent much of the last three decades trying to do just that, by writing articles with increasingly polemical titles (for example, "Please Don't Tell Me to Die Faster" and "Some Drugs Treat What Diets Could Prevent") and by creating interactive websites that attempt to teach consumers about their food choices. He grows meaner, crabbier, and more impatient every year, he says, but his message, for some reason, has not grabbed the public as strongly as the trans message or the cholesterol message has.

"The tissue is the issue," says Lands. "We can change our diets or we can spend billions of dollars a year to suppress omega-6 signaling, which is what aspirin, ibuprofen, acetaminophen, and the newer COX-2 inhibitors, Celebrex, Vioxx, and Bextra, do."

All the conditions for which we take these nonsteroidal anti-inflammatory drugs—conditions that include heart disease, stroke, arthritis, asthma, menstrual cramps, headaches, and tumor metastases—have excessive omega-6 signaling, he adds.

Another point that Lands never tires of making concerns serum cholesterol, the thing that worries Americans the most. Lands is adamant that serum cholesterol is nothing more than a risk factor associated with heart disease and cardiac death. It allows a degree of prediction about who will develop heart problems but has never been shown to actually cause these problems. (Much the same can be said of C-reactive protein, a risk factor that received a great deal of publicity in 2005.)

"We're in one of the most embarrassing times of science—like the Dark Ages," says Lands. "There's no plausible mechanism by which serum cholesterol could kill people, but we spend all our time and money on this target. By contrast, we've known how thromboxane can kill people since 1975."

TEN

WHERE HAVE ALL THE OMEGA-3s GONE?

Eat well of the cresses.

JOHN GRANGE, 1577

THE TIPPING POINT FOR MANY OF THE SCIENTISTS INVOLVED WITH omega-3 fatty acids was 1985. It was the year that researchers from around the world came to a conference in Washington, D.C., to present evidence and examine claims that eicosapentaenoic acid and DHA, two fats found in significant amounts in fish and fish-eating people, confer special benefits on human health.

The National Fisheries Institute, as well as the Department of Commerce and the National Institutes of Health (NIH), sponsored the conference, whose goal was to promote the consumption of fish and fish oil—which it did. But it also had the unintended effect of raising questions about the food supply, in general, and the amount of omega-6 fatty acids, the most effective competitors of omega-3, in the daily diet.

"This was one of the most exciting things I've ever participated in," says Howard Sprecher, the biochemist who worked out the pathway for the synthesis of DHA. "People made the connection that you could change the behavior of cells through nutritional means." "There were slides from American, Japanese,

German, and Danish populations that showed such striking changes in membranes and behavior," Artemis Simopoulos recalls; she is the physician who chaired the conference and was then the head of the NIH's Nutrition Coordinating Committee. "The idea emerged that the amount of omega-6s in the diet was too high."

William Lands was at that conference, as were Jørn Dyerberg and Alexander Leaf, the chief of medicine at Massachusetts General Hospital who would soon resign from his post to devote himself full-time to the study of omega-3 fatty acids. So was Norman Salem, a neurobiologist at NIH who studies the behavioral consequences associated with a deficiency of DHA, and William Connor, who has been researching the beneficial effects of fish and fish oils on blood lipids at the University of Oregon (and later at Oregon Health and Science University) since the 1970s.

All the participants arrived at the gathering with the belief that eating fish was beneficial because fish were endowed with large amounts of eicosapentaenoic acid and DHA. But they left with the understanding that eating fish might not be enough to prevent the diseases that were being linked to a diet that was low in omega-3 fats. The problem was that the tissues of Western populations were awash in omega-6s, fats that compete with the omega-3s.

"People walk around in seemingly good health with vastly differing amounts of omega-6 fats in their tissues," as Lands points out. "But the long-term disease consequences are enormous. They can have 78 percent of their HUFAs [highly unsaturated fatty acids] as omega-6s, as they do in the United States; 58 percent, as they do in Mediterranean countries like Italy and Greece; or 47 percent, as they do in Japan. Meanwhile mortality from heart disease goes up linearly with the increase in omega-6s, from 50 deaths per hundred thousand people in Japan, to 90 in Mediterranean countries, and 200 in the United States."

Where had these fats come from? Part of the answer was available at the time of the 1985 conference, in the form of tables detailing the fat content of a limited number of foods. These tables indicated that there were many more omega-6 fats than omega-3s in corn and soybeans, the primary ingredients of many processed foods and the feed choice of most farmers. They also showed that there are many more omega-6 fats in most vegetable oils and revealed a marked increase in omega-6 fats (and loss of omega-3 fats) when unprocessed vegetable oils, like soybean oil, are partially hydrogenated to make margarine.

Hydrogenation is a technique that was invented at the turn of the nineteenth century to turn vegetable oil into solid fat by eliminating all the double bonds in its fatty acid chains, thereby improving the stability of its flavor, broadening its use in cooking, and providing a low-cost alternative to butter and lard. Partial hydrogenation, as its name implies, eliminates just some of the double bonds in vegetable oils, resulting in a softer, less saturated product than does total hydrogenation.

Both linoleic and alpha linolenic acids are lost during total hydrogenation. But in partial hydrogenation, much more alpha linolenic is lost since it is more susceptible to both oxidation and hydrogenation. When this technique became the standard U.S. method for altering vegetable oils for use in processed foods, no one was concerned that this partial reduction of double bonds was at the expense of alpha linolenic acid, because no one knew that alpha linolenic acid was essential to human health. By the time this was recognized as a problem, the food industries had a lot at stake in maintaining the status quo.

If you talk to officials of these companies, as I have, they will tell you that vegetable oils and table fats have never been an important source of omega-3s; thus it doesn't matter that there are few of them in most vegetable oils and that they are eliminated during partial hydrogenation or selective breeding. What we need to do, according to industry spokespeople, is to eat more fish. While it is true that vegetable oils have never been an important source of omega-3s, we never had so many omega-6s in our diet before the twentieth century, when technological advances made it possible to squeeze every drop of oil out of seeds. Suggesting that our way out of this quandary is to eat more fish ignores the underlying competition between these fats.

But the complete answer to the question of where all the omega-6s had come from (and its flip side, the question of where all the omega-3s had gone) was fleshed out in the years following the conference with studies of the trends in food supplies and with a more complete analysis of the omega-6 and omega-3 content of different foods—and of foods produced in different ways (for example, whether animals were free-range or were fed in feed lots). These expanded food tables and food surveys showed clearly what the participants of that 1985 conference had begun to suspect. "Our diet is greatly out of whack," as Simopoulos puts it bluntly, and many of our agricultural and food-processing techniques promote the inclusion of omega-6s in our diets (and tissues) at the expense of omega-3s.

The United States Department of Agriculture (USDA) has been keeping track of some (not all) of the fats in the food supply ever since 1909, and its records show that per capita intake of linoleic acid, the parent omega-6 fatty acid, has been steadily increasing: it went up from about 7 grams per day in the years 1909 to 1913 to more than 25 grams, or about 2 tablespoons of the stuff, in 1985. Part of this rise is due to the response of consumers to concerns about their cholesterol levels and to advice to increase their intake of polyunsaturated fats. Since the 1960s, when it was widely recognized that polyunsaturated vegetable oils not only are cholesterol-free, like all plant oils, but also reduce serum cholesterol, there has been a fourfold increase in the use of vegetable oil–based salad and cooking oils. And part is due to the increase in processed foods in the American diet, for linoleic acid is the main polyunsaturate in processed foods.

"Processed foods and alpha linolenic acid are incompatible," Bob Brown of Frito-Lay told me in a telephone interview. "Some foods that have a short shelf life can stand a certain amount of alpha linolenic acid, but it is ten times less stable than linoleic acid, so it cannot be used in processed foods." Gary List, a chemist with the USDA, agrees: "Any product with significant amounts of alpha linolenic acid has a stability problem."

The USDA did not track calories from alpha linolenic acid during this same time period, but it did track saturated fats. Per capita intake of these fats has also been increasing during those same years, though far less dramatically (rising from 52 grams per person per day in 1909–13 to about 58 in 1985). Saturated fats, as a percentage of total fat, have fallen, from about 42 percent to 34 percent. According to the lipid hypothesis, these changes should have resulted in a significant fall in the incidence of heart disease in the United States. But they haven't. The only thing that has changed about heart disease in this time has been a significant drop in the mortality rate, attributable to improved methods of treatment.

In some countries, Israel in particular, both the incidence of *and* mortality from heart disease have gone up with rising intake of linoleic acid, of which Israel consumes more per capita than any other country in the world (more than 30 grams a day). This is a trend known as the Israeli paradox, but it seems paradoxical only to those who believe in the benefits of polyunsaturated fatty acids, as a general class, and make no distinction between omega-3s and omega-6s. Israelis eat less animal fat and cholesterol and fewer calories than Americans, but they have comparable rates of heart disease, obesity, diabetes, and many cancers. They have an ideal diet, as far as the American food pyramid is concerned, but far from ideal health. "Israeli Jews may be regarded as a population-based dietary experiment of the effect of a high omega-6 PUFA [polyunsaturated fatty acid] diet," the authors of a paper on the Israeli paradox conclude. Until recently, they add, this diet was widely recommended.

Trends in the food supplies are very revealing, and I will come back to them in this chapter. But perhaps the most interesting perspective on how diets have been changing comes from a research tack taken by Artemis Simopoulos after the 1985 conference. The food tables that were available at the time of the conference listed the content of very few green vegetables. But those figures—for spinach, leeks, lettuce, kale, and broccoli—were surprising to Simopoulos. These green leafy vegetables, it appeared, have significant amounts of fat. Not as much fat as seeds, grains, or the flesh of fish and fowl, certainly, but more fat than most people would have ever expected. And what fats they do have are mostly alpha linolenic acid, from the omega-3 family.

"All grains are high in omega-6s, and all green plants are high in omega-3s," says Simopoulos today. This same realization led her in 1985 to hypothesize that a diet rich in greens might also be a significant source of the omega-3 fats. Simopoulos, who was born in Greece but attended college and medical school in the United States, remembered how the animals ate in her native country. She recalled how goats scrambled up the hills to browse on bushes and how chickens scratched for insects and wild greens, and she wondered if those wild greens make a difference in the eggs, milk, cheese, and meat that is eaten in Greece, a country with very little heart disease. The Greeks are also a fish-eating population with a high intake of olive oil, two aspects of the diet that are usually given all the credit for the low rate of heart disease, but Simopoulos became curious about the role of greens.

Simopoulos began by testing purslane, one of the most common wild greens in Greece (and many other countries). She was amazed to find that this ordinary plant, a weed in most of the world's eyes, has an alpha linolenic acid content four times that of cultivated spinach (about 0.4 grams per 100 grams). Purslane is not a cold-adapted plant like some other greens full of omega-3s, such as rapeseed (canola), spinach, and aquatic plants. It is not for that reason that it is full of omega-3s. Rather, botanists suspect, its high level of omega-3s works to compensate for light damage, since purslane grows in intense sunlight. (There you have it: something else about fats that has only recently been learned. Linseed, or flaxseed, is another plant that is high in alpha linolenic acid and grows in a hot climate.)

Then Simopoulos tested a Greek egg, which came from a Greek chicken that had feasted on purslane, insects, and only small amounts of corn. She found that this egg was extremely rich (1.78 g per 100 g) in all the omega-3 fatty acids, including DHA and eicosapentaenoic acid—as rich as, if not richer than, many species of fish. One hundred grams of farmed Atlantic salmon have about the same amount of omega-3 fatty acids. Sardines have more, and anchovies have less. An egg purchased in an American supermarket, in contrast, had a tenth the omega-3 fatty acids as its Greek counterpart. The American egg had come from a factory-raised chicken, fed largely on corn.

In time, other researchers would find the same pattern in free-range versus grain-fed beef, lamb, and pork (and in the milk and cheese from these animals), and botanists would clarify the role played by alpha linolenic and linoleic acids in plants, the source of both these essential fats. Alpha linolenic acid is the fat that plants use in the membranes of their chloroplasts (the thylacoid membrane), the fat that surrounds their complex machinery of photosynthesis and enables plants to capture photons and turn them into carbohydrates.

Linoleic acid, in contrast, is a kind of storage fat for plants, to be turned into alpha linolenic acid as needed by a special desaturase enzyme that only plants have. It is found in highest concentrations in seeds and has no other function in plants than to be the precursor of alpha linolenic acid. It is less prone to oxidation than its omega-3 cousin, as we know, and thus can be safely stored until photosynthesis is necessary at the moment of germination.

And so it seemed to Simopoulos that one of the most important ways that the diets of Western countries have been changing is that Western populations are consuming more seeds, and the fats of seeds, and fewer greens, and the fats of greens. This shift has been taking place since the beginnings of agriculture, she realized, when cultivated crops began replacing foraged foods, but sped up greatly in the past century as seed oils became a significant source of food calories and as alpha linolenic acid was eliminated from foods in order to improve their shelf life. The former development has resulted from advances that have made it economical to extract more of the oil from seeds; the latter, from the hydrogenation and partial hydrogenation of oils, as I've mentioned, and from selective breeding of plants.

Plant biologists have been selecting for low alpha linolenic varieties of soybeans since the 1980s with the goals of improving stability and cutting down on hydrogenation costs. Now they are looking for similar forms of rapeseeds. Low alpha linolenic varieties of plants like spinach have probably been *unknowingly* selected for over the centuries in order to reduce the tendency of green leaves to spoil.

It was also becoming clear to Simopoulos why fish had become so important to human health. Not only are fish endowed with larger amounts of DHA and eicosapentaenoic acid than terrestrial animals (thus enabling fish to see and move around in their dim, cold, watery environments), but they are also some of the last wild foods in the human diet. Most fish eat the wild foods—the algae, plankton, and other fish—that they have always eaten and that are full of the fats found naturally in leaves. Phytoplankton is the largest mass of photosynthetic machinery on the planet, and it contributes the largest amount of alpha linolenic acid. (A number of alga and plankton species also produce DHA and eicosapentaenoic acid, as I've already mentioned, thereby adding to the nutritional importance of the fish that consume them.)

Fish raised in aquaculture farms have more grains in their diet, it is true, but fortunately for humans, fish are much less tolerant of a reduced intake of omega-3s than are land animals. Their diets can't be greatly altered without a significant increase in mortality. Fish differ from warm-blooded animals not because they require omega-3s, as investigators first thought, but because they require so much of them. They need to have an absolute minimum of 1 percent of their calories as omega-3s, versus 0.5 percent in warm-blooded animals. Because fish have this higher requirement, it's no coincidence that the first animals to show a clear omega-3 deficiency were trout that were being fed corn oil as their only source of fats. These trout exhibited poor growth, fin erosion, high mortality, and a "fainting" or shock syndrome never before observed: a loss of consciousness if the fish are handled or their tank is given a sharp blow.

Simopoulos was one of the first people to compare the fats in wild and cultivated greens, much as Michael Crawford was the first to compare the fats in wild and domesticated animals. Their research has led to the large numbers of omega-3 supplemented foods—eggs, milk, and meats—that are available in many grocery stores today. These foods are more expensive than their unsupplemented counterparts, but they lack a medical price tag—the billions of dollars that Americans spend to suppress omega-6 signaling each year. The point is not to "turn the clock back" to a time when animals foraged for themselves, says Crawford, "but to move forward with new ideas."

Simopoulos's work has also led to the understanding, slow in coming, that most of the omega-3s in our diets and tissues ultimately come from green leaves and most of the omega-6s come from seeds, a recognition that is fundamental to sound advice about eating and nutrition. Fish consumption counts, but our problems are probably caused not by a lack of fish in our diets but by an overconsumption of seed oils and an underconsumption of greens. Understanding this requires an appreciation of the rivalry between fatty acids.

According to food disappearance studies, the amount of long-chain omega-6 fatty acids (arachidonic acid) in the American diet is very small (less than one-tenth of a percent of energy intake), as small as or smaller than the amount of long-chain omega-3 fatty acids (DHA and eicosapentaenoic acid). Yet our tissues are full of these stormy, troublesome (but essential) fats. How did this happen?

There is only one way: they enter the diet, and our bodies, as linoleic acid and overwhelm the preferences of Holman's enzymes (the desaturases and elongases) to become arachidonic acid. Data for the United States indicate that Americans consumed between 11 and 16 grams of linoleic acid per day during the years 1989–91 and about 1 to 2 grams of alpha linolenic acid. At that ratio, only about 15 percent of the alpha linolenic acid is converted to DHA and eicosapentaenoic acid. At lower ratios, the conversion rate is much higher. The best conversion occurs at a ratio of 2.3:1.

More evidence for the idea that it is not the fish we are *not* eating that is our problem, but the oils we *are* eating, comes from observations and studies of faraway populations.

In the decades since Dyerberg and Bang first visited the west coast of Greenland, the diet of the Eskimos has been changing—and not for the better. Dyerberg and Bang made the inhabitants of the settlement of Igdlorssuit famous with their studies on bleeding time and diet, but that did not stop those inhabitants from adopting many of the same foods that Westerners eat, including vegetable oils and packaged foods. "We always told you it was the seal that made us healthy," Eskimos were heard bragging after the studies began making headlines. But by 1988, rates of heart disease in Eskimo and Danish populations were very similar; by 2003, there was no difference between the two groups. Yet the Eskimos in Igdlorssuit still consume large quantities of seal and fish, more seafood than any Western populations. The explanation for the change in heart disease is that they now consume large amounts of other fats that compete with the fats in fish and seal.

Ralph Holman succinctly expresses the key to this life-and-death issue: "Metabolism is going to happen whether we like it or not." In other words, linoleic acid is going to be turned into arachidonic acid no matter how much fish a person is eating, as long as that person is consuming large amounts of omega-6 vegetable oils and not enough greens.

A second population that is very revealing is that of Enugu, Nigeria, an inland town where little fish is consumed. In the 1960s, Holman had a postdoctoral student from Nigeria in his lab; and in the 1980s, long after this student had returned to Africa, he sent Holman blood samples from thirty-eight of his compatriots. Using his gas-liquid chromatograph to examine the fatty acid profiles of these healthy Nigerians from the town of Enugu, Holman found that their omega-3 content was higher than in any other population he had studied—about twice as high as his Minnesota controls. These Nigerians didn't eat very much fish, but they did eat a lot of greens and no high omega-6 vegetable oils. The major source of their dietary fat is fresh palm oil, which is high in saturated fats; and saturated fats, as Holman knew, are poor competitors of the omega-3s.

"This is exactly what we demonstrated three decades ago in this laboratory," says Holman. And it translates to a simple piece of nutritional advice on which all the omega-3 researchers agree. "You have to reduce your omega-6s if you want to get any benefit from omega-3s," warns Alexander Leaf. Bill Lands echoes his sentiments: "Eat more omega-3s and less omega-6s. That's a direction you can go in with certainty."

I wish I could tell you that this is the same advice that the American public is being given, but recognition of this research, and its profound implications, has been slow in coming, especially in the United States. To be sure, 1985 may have been the tipping point for scientists involved with omega-3 fatty acids, and the year marked the beginning of numerous studies into the role that omega-6 fats play in the promotion of certain cancers, including breast, prostate, and colon cancer, and into the benefits of omega-3s in treating psychological disorders such as depression and postpartum depression, attention deficit disorder, and bipolar disorder. But it was also the beginning of a large and growing disconnect between the scientists who study these fats and the government and medical organizations that make recommendations about diet and health.

As of their most recent revision in 2005, the USDA's dietary guidelines, the cornerstone of federal nutrition policy, do not distinguish between the different families of essential fatty acids.

Fish is mentioned as containing "a certain type of polyunsaturated fatty acid (omega-3) that is under study because of a possible association with a decreased risk for heart disease in certain people." But the emphasis is on the importance of lowering saturated fats and cholesterol in order to reduce blood cholesterol, and all kinds of "unsaturated fats," they say, "reduce blood cholesterol when they replace saturated fats in the diet." As of the year 2004, the American Heart Association also does not distinguish between the two families of fats. "Polyunsaturated and monounsaturated fats are the two unsaturated fats," the AHA's website states. "They're found primarily in oils from plants."

The Institute of Medicine of the National Academy of Sciences is an exception in recognizing the different roles of omega-6 and omega-3 fatty acids, but the adequate intakes it sets for each (12 to 17 grams for omega-6s, and 1.1 to 1.6 grams daily for omega-3s) result in a ratio between the two families of about 10 to 1—very close to the current ratio in the United States, which is associated with a high rate of disease. This is much higher than the ratio recommended by Sweden (5:1) or Japan (2:1), two other countries that have established guidelines. While no one knows what the optimal ratio in the diet is for these two families of fats, it is thought that humans evolved under conditions in which they were about equal. As we've learned, the body gets the most DHA and eicosapentaenoic acid out of alpha linolenic acid when the ratio is about 2.3:1.

The scientists who work with omega-3s have different ideas as to why it is taking government and health organizations so long to digest this new information about fats. For Simopoulos, "It's a question of economics. The edible oils industry is a very powerful lobby and soybeans and corn are some of our major commodities." When I asked Alexander Leaf if his finding that DHA could prevent fatal arrhythmia, the tendency of heart cells to develop abnormal rhythms, was readily accepted, he replied,

"Oh, hell, no. I had a terrible time getting those papers even published though no one had any criticisms about their methodology. The cardiologists and pharmaceutical industry don't like to hear this. They have a multibillion-dollar business going on and they don't want someone coming along and saying, 'All you have to do is change what you put on your plate a little bit and you can avoid all these problems.'"

Norman Salem, who has made it his lifelong quest to know how DHA functions in the nervous system, is less cynical but no less urgent. "It's a slow process and will take time," he says. "People have a hard time giving up the assumption that the way they eat now is not the way they have always eaten—nor is it the healthiest way."

Most scientists agree that the cholesterol story has dominated medical thinking, and some acknowledge that the science of fatty acids isn't the easiest to follow, with names and family trees more complicated than those in a Russian novel; ever-expanding plot lines (a growing list of the diseases in which omega-6s and omega-3s play a part); and no clear villain, since humans require even more linoleic acid than they do alpha linolenic acid. "We have to be careful with our recommendations so that people don't start avoiding omega-6 fats," Jørn Dyerberg reminds me. "It's a matter of balance and of understanding how out of balance most diets and populations have become."

Then there are concerns about advising individuals to consume more fish (the best known form of omega-3s) when the contaminants in fish can pose significant health problems. Plus there is the unavoidable fact, the elephant in the living room, that organizations will have to retract some of their previous dietary advice in order to correct the imbalance of omega-6 and omega-3 fats. Reducing saturated fat has been a goal for several decades, and there is no question that large amounts of saturated

The Fat Matters

Cooking and Salad Oils	Ratio of Omega-6s to Omega-3s
Flaxseed or linseed	0.2 : 1
Canola	2 : 1
Canola (for light frying)[a]	3 : 1
Walnut	5 : 1
Soybean	7 : 1
Wheat germ	8 : 1
Butter	9 : 1
Lard	10 : 1
Olive	12 : 1
Hydrogenated soybean	13 : 1
High oleic sunflower	19 : 1
Corn	46 : 1
Palm	46 : 1
Sesame	137 : 1
Less than 60% linoleic sunflower	200 : 1
Cottonseed	259 : 1

SOURCE: USDA Nutrient Data Laboratory data, available from the USDA Agricultural Research Service at www.ars.usda.gov.

NOTE: To put these numbers into some sort of context, boiled New Zealand spinach has a ratio of 0.2:1; baked halibut, 0.3:1. Safflower oil is not included in the table because its total lack of omega-3s, according to the USDA data, would make the "ratio" an absurd "infinity to 1." Other sources suggest a ratio of about 115:1. All these ratios are approximate, remember, since the fatty acid content of fats and oils changes with temperature, season, breeding, processing, and, in the case of butter and lard, what the cow and pig ate.

[a] A modified form of canola oil with less alpha linolenic acid.

fats in the diet present a problem. But saturated fats are poorer at competing with omega-3s than omega-6s, so small amounts of saturated fats are better than large amounts of omega-6s.

As of January 2006, information about trans fats has joined data on saturated fats on food labels in the United States. But this change won't lead to healthier eating unless consumers understand the trade-off they will be asked to make in order to have foods that are both trans-free and low in saturates: a higher mono-unsaturate content or a higher omega-6 content. And they must understand that reducing trans and saturated fat is not enough to produce good health: they still need a source of omega-3s. (Perhaps surprisingly, there isn't even a clear scientific consensus on the negative effects of trans fats; much of the push to add trans as well as saturated fats to labels has come from the producers of saturated fats, who felt that they were being unfairly singled out. Recall that the trans fats in vegetable oils result from the partial hydrogenation process that selectively eliminates omega-3s, so only very well-controlled studies are able to distinguish between effects caused by the presence of trans fats in the diet and those caused by the lack of omega-3s. That said, trans fats are less fluid and flexible than cis fats, and they do compete for positions in cell membranes—so it can't hurt to avoid them. But they don't play the same important roles as omega-3s and omega-6s.)

There are ways out of this conundrum, but they require backpedaling on the question of saturated fats. European food producers have been using the technique of interesterification to produce oils that are stable *and* contain a certain amount of alpha linolenic acid, but there is a rub: these oils have more saturated fat than many of the vegetable oils currently available in the United States. In order for these new oils, formed by rearranging the fatty acids on triglycerides, to become acceptable, our government would have to back down on its stance on these fats.

It would have to admit that maybe it didn't know as much as it said it did about the role that fats play in a healthy diet. Vegetable oil producers would have to make the change from hydrogenation to interesterification technology.

Other remedies that might be easier for officials and the public to swallow include supplementation of foods with fish, flax, and alga oils; recommendations to increase consumption of fish and greens; mandatory enrichment of eggs; and the development of high omega-3 oils through other means, including selective breeding and genetic engineering. But sooner or later, the public is going to have to be presented with the whole picture about fats, complicated as it may be. Given the growing number of diseases that are being associated with an imbalance of the essential fats—not just heart disease, cancers, depression, immune disorders, and arthritis but also obesity and diabetes, as the next chapter will show—it should probably be sooner.

ELEVEN

THE SPEED OF LIFE

The fire of life seems to burn brighter in some than others.

D. S. MILLER, AMERICAN PHYSIOLOGIST

READERS WITH A PHILOSOPHICAL BENT MAY ALREADY BE WONDER-
ing why the fats of leaves and the fats of seeds would have such
different effects on human health. They may already have hypothesized that the disparity has something to do with the fact
that these fats are markers of the changing seasons—as good as,
if not better than, light and temperature. Once incorporated into
an animal's cell membranes, they might help an animal prepare
for the future: for periods of activity and reproduction, when the
fats of leaves are abundant, and periods of hunkering down and
survival, when the fats of seeds are more plentiful.

These preparations could be accomplished and coordinated
by signals of the different fatty acids (as eicosanoids) and by
changes in the membranes themselves, since the membrane is the
medium in which many enzymes and proteins work, the air in
which they breathe. Not all the membranes would have to
change with changes in seasons and food supply. Some might be
protected from change, as it seems the membranes of the cells of
the brain and nervous system are protected. Humans would have
benefited from these seasonal changes in their membranes when

they were foraging animals, but we ran into trouble when the seasonal became permanent and we began eating high omega-6 diets year-round. This idea makes a great deal of sense, but it is just an idea, the germ of a hypothesis. It's an idea that only became possible, though, as researchers have learned to distinguish between omega-6s and omega-3s, the two families of fats that humans and other animals cannot make from scratch. Until recently, most researchers grouped the two families together, calling them all polyunsaturated fatty acids, or PUFAs (pronounced *poofas*). Prior to the 1960s, few had the means to distinguish between them.

Times have changed, though, and nature is giving up its secrets to those who know the names of these different fatty acids and who control for them in their experiments. Among these researchers is Lawrence Rudel at Wake Forest University School of Medicine, who found that omega-3 fatty acids, but not omega-6s, decrease atherosclerosis in his experimental animals by creating more fluid cholesterol droplets and increasing the rate of cholesterol hydrolysis and departure from cells (much as Ralph Holman has been suggesting since the 1950s). And Leonard Sauer and Robert Dauchy at the Bassett Research Institute in Cooperstown, N.Y., who find it easy to grow tumors in their experimental animals when those animals are being fed a diet rich in corn oil (linoleic acid), but almost impossible when the corn oil is replaced with fish oil.

And Gregory Florant, who studies hibernation, and the cues that trigger it, in the yellow-bellied marmot, a relative of the common hamster and a denizen of Colorado, where Florant works. The role of fats in hibernation was a great puzzle to researchers when they grouped all the polyunsaturates together. No consistent pattern could be found in either the tissues of hibernating animals or the foods they ate. But as soon as Florant

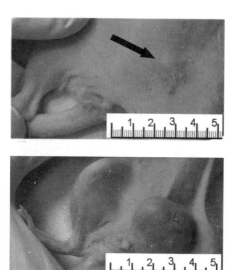

FIGURE 7 Tumor growth. Human breast tumors were implanted in both these nude rats, but the tumor in the animal on the bottom is growing much faster than the one in the animal on the top. The only difference is their diet. Fifteen days after implantation, the top animal was switched from a 5% corn oil diet (the control) to a 5% omega-3 diet. Leonard Sauer and Robert Dauchy at the Bassett Research Institute in Cooperstown, N.Y., have run this same experiment using many different lines of human and rat tumors; each time, their results have been similar. If they start the rats out on a 5% omega-3 diet (rather than switching to it after 15 days), they can't even get the implantations to take. Photo by and courtesy of Leonard Sauer and Robert Dauchy.

distinguished between omega-3s and omega-6s, he saw a clear and very revealing pattern.

When Florant fed his marmots a diet rich in linseed oil, a diet with an alpha linolenic content close to that of their natural summer diet, they did not go into hibernation when Florant put them in a cold room in total darkness in October. They continued eating throughout the winter. They were unlike any other marmots that Florant had ever observed and unlike marmots that were fed a high omega-6 laboratory chow. The latter stopped feeding when Florant put them under winter conditions even though food was still available and even though they weighed the same as the experimental marmots. The omega-6 marmots fell asleep on schedule.

Florant attributes this striking difference in behavior to changes in the eicosanoids or prostaglandins produced by the marmots. But nothing in his study rules out an explanation based on more general changes in membranes due to diets that are rich in one or the other type of fat. These effects are the subject of ongoing research by a group of scientists in Australia and are the best evidence yet for the idea that there are profound differences between diets and tissues full of omega-6s and omega-3s, differences that slow our bodies down and speed them up. To explain their findings, the Australian scientists have developed what they call the pacemaker theory or the leaky membrane hypothesis.

In order to do justice to this theory, and the considerable research that lies behind it, I should start at the beginning. In the late 1970s, a young comparative biologist at the University of Wollongong, an Australian who had recently finished a postdoctoral fellowship at Cornell University in New York, asked a seemingly simple question. What, Tony Hulbert wondered, determines an animal's metabolic rate, the speed at which it burns fuel?

Metabolic rates, the cost of living during normal activity, vary greatly across the animal spectrum, as Hulbert knew, from the slow plodding of reptiles to the high speeds of small mammals. They differ by a factor of at least forty, changing with the size of animals and their life spans (smaller animals have faster metabolic rates and shorter lives). That much was known about these large differences in fuel consumption, but surprisingly little else until Hulbert decided to explore the question. He would use the resources he had at hand: the great diversity of animal life in Australia.

Hulbert and a graduate student, Paul Else, began by comparing a desert lizard, the central netted dragon, to a local mouse. These were two animals of the same size but with a sevenfold difference in metabolic rate (even when kept at the same temperature, the lizard's preferred temperature of 37°C, or about 99°F). They found that the activities of these animals' cells—production of ATP (adenosine triphosphate) and consumption of oxygen, for example—vary in the same way that their metabolic rate does. They are linked, in other words, and change in unison.

Hulbert and Else went on to compare marsupials and other mammals, amphibians like the cane toad (an introduced species that is one of the banes of Australia's existence) and other reptiles, and found the same thing. The activity of every cell function they could measure was high in speedy animals and low in slow ones, scaling up and down with metabolic rate like a set of Russian dolls. And yet, as the Australian scientists also determined, the cells of all these different animals were remarkably alike in their protein content. They had about the same number of enzymes and other working parts.

This finding surprised the two researchers: they had expected, as almost anyone would have, that harder-working cells would contain more working components. But that wasn't the case. So it must be that the enzymes in speedier animals work harder, they thought, and they tested this idea with an elegant series of crossover experiments. Since the proteins and enzymes they were looking at are embedded in membranes (where most of a cell's activities take place), they put the proteins from toad membranes into rat membranes and vice versa. The results of these experiments turned their attention away from enzymes and other proteins and toward fats, the fats or phospholipids in membranes. For what Hulbert and Else found was that rat proteins slow down in toad membranes and toad proteins speed up in rat membranes.

The total amount of fat was also the same in the membranes of these different animals: what differed, Hulbert and Else found, was the degree of unsaturation of the fatty acid chains—that is, the number of double bonds. Except in the brain, where the fats of all animals were remarkably constant (as Michael Crawford was the first to observe), fatty acids in slow animals such as lizards and toads were more·saturated than fatty acids in speedier animals. The fats of large, slow mammals were more saturated and contained more omega-6 fatty acids than the fats of small, fast mammals like the mouse, which contained more DHA. The fats of high-speed animals like the hummingbird were loaded with DHA.

Those high amounts of DHA resulted, as Hulbert and Else went on to discover, in leakier membranes—membranes that sodium molecules and protons find easier to cross and in which membrane pumps (in the form of proteins embedded in the membrane) must work harder in order to maintain the gradients across them. Those gradients are necessary to drive the cell's reactions, and maintaining them constitutes the largest portion of an animal's cost of living. "Warm-blooded mammals and cold-blooded reptiles have the same number of pumps in their membranes," says Hulbert, "but the pumps in warm-blooded animals have to work that much harder because the membranes are that much leakier, which leads to a higher metabolic rate." And while leaky membranes and harder-working pumps might not sound like such a good thing to have (we all know what happens to engines when they run constantly), leaky, fluid membranes allow all of a cell's reactions to take place faster, speeding up not just proton and sodium pumps but also nerve impulses, signal reception, and muscle contractions, including those of the heart.

"A membrane needs to be cohesive enough to be a barrier, but fluid and disordered enough so that the proteins, enzymes, and receptors that are embedded in it can move around freely and do the things they need to do," explains Burton Litman, an NIH researcher who studies the role of DHA in vision. "DHA gives membranes that degree of disorder." Another NIH researcher credits DHA with creating a membrane with "tumultuous disorder and behavior that is almost liquid-like."

Hulbert and Else agree, for they have found it is the DHA content of membranes that correlates most closely with an animal's metabolic rate. It is the concentration of this highly unsaturated fatty acid that scales up and down with body size and all the activities of an animal's cells, including an animal's heart rate. DHA has six double bonds, as we know, adding a kind of flexibility or looseness to the membrane, thereby providing room for enzymes to maneuver and proteins to twist and turn. The last double bond, just three carbons in from the end of the tail, is particularly important, adding elbow room to the very middle of the membrane.

Recent computer simulations and nuclear magnetic resonance studies present "an image of DHA thrashing about in the hydrocarbon core of the membrane," Hulbert writes. "Such molecular movement of DHA in a membrane bilayer suggests that it will likely speed up, in a relatively non-specific manner, many processes catalyzed by membrane proteins."

"What we see with DHA is a rapid interconversion between an almost uncountable number of different conformations," says Scott Feller, a chemist who uses X-ray scattering and nuclear magnetic resonance techniques to study the behavior of DHA. "A saturated chain will almost always be aligned perpendicular to the membrane, but DHA can go from an elongated, perpendicular position to one where its tail is almost sticking out of the membrane." This is the equivalent, as another researcher told me, of the oil and vinegar in salad dressing combining, separating, and recombining on their own. Exactly how this high-speed flip-flopping speeds up the proteins in membranes researchers are only just beginning to discover, but some describe DHA as a molecular spring.

The number of different positions that unsaturated fatty acids can get into drops off dramatically with each double bond, which is probably why the five double-bonded molecule that our bodies make when we are deficient in omega-3s (an elongated and desaturated version of the omega-6 fatty acid arachidonic acid) leads to neurological and developmental problems, as researchers have clearly found.

"You couldn't be an astronaut or a fighter pilot if you were raised on an omega-3-deficient diet," declares Litman, who has found that rhodopsin, the protein responsible for our ability to sense light, is much more active in membranes rich in DHA. Michael Crawford emphasizes omega-3's role in the brain. "Nature's enigmatic choice of high DHA levels for neural membranes is conserved across a broad range of species," he says. "The brain is exquisitely sensitive to slight differences in fatty acids."

Hulbert and Else's work is leading to a new appreciation of the role of DHA and of increasing unsaturation in membranes. But these two researchers are also the first to point out that DHA's flexibility, its ability to thrash about and rise to the surface of membranes, does not come without a cost. DHA's varying concentration in membranes probably explains why the animals with the highest metabolic rates have the shortest lives, an association first observed about a century ago. Because the six double bonds of DHA are susceptible to attack by oxygen molecules, animals with the most highly unsaturated membranes will generate the most free radicals and will age faster and die sooner than those whose membranes are more saturated.

This may sound like a good reason *not* to eat greens and fish. But remember: at the same time that those animals are accumulating free radicals, their hearts are beating faster, their minds are thinking more clearly, their muscles are moving more quickly, and their bodies are burning more fuel. The Japanese currently have the longest life expectancy *and* the highest omega-3 consumption of any living population of humans. They are also among the leanest, which puts the finding that Americans who are somewhat overweight have longer lives, reported with glee in April 2005, into a more international context. The pacemaker theory would predict that humans who weigh more and have slower metabolisms would live longer, but only in an environment like that of the United States, where medicines that compensate for the drawbacks of that extra weight are widely available.

Metabolism, life span, and health are tightly linked, as this research is showing; and they are controlled by genetic factors (variations in many enzymes, including those that are responsible for desaturating and elongating fatty acids and inserting them into membranes), as well as environmental and dietary ones. Among those dietary factors are the amounts of omega-6s and omega-3s that animals eat.

"Oils ain't oils," as Leonard Storlien likes to say. Storlien is an obesity expert who was perhaps the first person to see the implications of Hulbert and Else's pacemaker theory for problems associated with energy balance and obesity. "If you have a person running at a metabolic rate that is 40 percent of someone else," observes this Canadian-born researcher, who moved to Australia to teach and earn his Ph.D., "you would have a profound predisposition for obesity."

Storlien was a researcher at the Garvan Institute of Medical Research in Darlinghurst in the late 1980s when he first heard of Hulbert and Else's work. He had been using an animal model to study insulin resistance, a decrease in the ability of tissues to remove glucose from the blood and the precursor to type 2 diabetes in humans, and was looking for an explanation for an unusual finding in his lab. Why did fish oil, he wondered, prevent his experimental rats from developing this condition, which causes both high blood glucose levels and a decrease in energy expenditure? Storlien had already found that rats do develop insulin resistance on diets that were rich in either saturated fats or omega-6s. But fish oil was different, as he learned in the mid-1980s. It protected against both insulin resistance and obesity.

Storlien decided to try these experiments after reading about Dyerberg and Bang's trips to Greenland and picking up on a little-noticed comment in one of their first papers. "Not a single established case of diabetes mellitus is known at present in the population of the Umanak district," they noted in 1971. "This disease is extremely rare in Greenlanders in general."

Most people who followed Dyerberg and Bang's work were interested in the Eskimos' low rate of heart disease, as we know. But because Storlien was concerned about the skyrocketing numbers of people in countries such as Australia and the United States with type 2 diabetes, or non-insulin-dependent diabetes mellitus (NIDDM), a condition very common in obese people, this sentence leaped out at him. The dogma at the time was that high-fat diets promoted obesity and diabetes, as well as heart disease, and Storlien himself had found that saturated fats in the diets of rats produce a rapid and profound insulin resistance. But the Eskimos ate a diet that was high in fat and had none of these problems. What was the difference, he wondered? Perhaps it had something to do with polyunsaturated fats.

I use the word *polyunsaturated* judiciously. By the mid-1980s, when Storlien was embarking on these experiments, Dyerberg and Bang already knew that all polyunsaturates are not alike. But that's not something they knew in 1971, at the time they wrote the comment that piqued Storlien's interest. So when Storlien chose a polyunsaturated fat to test this idea, he picked the polyunsaturated fat most readily available to him in Australia in 1986: safflower oil, the same vegetable oil that had led to Shawna Strobel's omega-3 deficiency. "In some ways it was sheer laziness to use safflower oil," says Storlien today. "It was easy to get and easy to mix in the diet."

Storlien put a group of rats on this high omega-6 polyunsaturated diet and they, too, quickly developed insulin resistance (as compared to rats on a high-carbohydrate diet). This new result also fit in well with the dogma that high-fat diets promote diabetes. But it didn't fit in with the Eskimos' low rate of diabetes. So Storlien reread all of Dyerberg and Bang's papers, and he began thinking about eicosapentaenoic acid. Was there really something unusual about this polyunsaturated fatty acid, something that protected the Eskimos against both heart disease and diabetes?

Storlien then gave fish oil (containing both eicosapentaenoic acid and DHA) to a new group of rats and found that it did indeed prevent those rats from developing insulin resistance. All he had to do was to replace just 6 percent of the linoleic acid in the diet with long-chain omega-3 fats; rats were then able to maintain their ability to remove glucose from the blood, though their total fat intake remained the same.

Storlien's earlier work had been well received by the scientists in his field, but this new finding generated an enormous amount of flak from what he has come to call "the low-fat mafia." "I got e-mails saying, 'This can't possibly be true. It couldn't work in humans,'" Storlien told me during one of our several telephone interviews. "At conferences, people would stand up and say, 'Everyone knows that fish oil deteriorates blood glucose,' even though that was not true in well-controlled studies. What helped my case was that there were a number of cross-sectional, epidemiological studies coming out at the same time, and they showed that an increased fish intake is associated with a reduced incidence of diabetes."

Storlien was searching the scientific literature for mechanisms that could explain the effects of fish and fish oil when he heard about Hulbert and Else's leaky membrane hypothesis and immediately saw its implications for understanding the cluster of diseases surrounding energy balance and insulin resistance in humans—the so-called metabolic syndrome, or syndrome X, as it is widely known. Leaky membranes increase energy expenditure by increasing the amount of work that membrane pumps need to do, as Hulbert and Else had shown. Such membranes might also, Storlien realized as he read their work, increase the effectiveness, or sensitivity, of the insulin receptor, which is a membrane-embedded protein. He and the two comparative biologists have been collaborating ever since.

Hulbert was already at the University of Wollongong when Storlien joined the faculty in 1994 to head the department of biomedical sciences. One of his first decisions was to bring back Paul Else, who had finished his Ph.D. and was teaching at another university. The three of them formed the nucleus of the Metabolic Research Center at the University of Wollongong and have written a number of theoretical papers together, as well as pursuing their independent lines of inquiry into the role of membranes in metabolism and health.

Hulbert and Else looked at a wide variety of birds, for example, and found the same relationship of DHA to body mass and metabolism they had found in reptiles and mammals. (DHA makes up only 6 percent of the phospholipids in the muscle membranes of the 70-pound emu, but 70 percent in the tiny, speedy hummingbird.) Storlien and a group of researchers, some from the NIH, studied the human population with the highest incidence of type 2 diabetes in the world, the Pima Indians of Arizona, and found half the amount of DHA in the phospholipids of their skeletal muscle as in a group of Australian, largely Caucasian, men (1.2 percent versus 2.5 percent). Skeletal muscle is the major site of glucose uptake in the body, and this difference in DHA content was closely correlated with the Indians' insulin resistance.

Storlien and these same researchers also found a probable genetic basis for this decrease in DHA *and* for the susceptibility of the Pima Indians to diabetes when they looked at the activity of the enzymes that desaturate and elongate fatty acids. These are Holman's enzymes, the enzymes that turn alpha linolenic acid and linoleic acid into the longer-chain HUFAs. And the activity of one of them, the delta-5 desaturase, was greatly reduced in the Pima population, resulting in less arachidonic acid, as well as less DHA and eicosapentaenoic acid, in their tissues.

The change in the activity of this enzyme also suggested a possible mechanism for another well-known hypothesis: the thrifty gene hypothesis, which was first proposed by the physician James Neel in 1962 to explain the high incidence of diabetes and heart disease in populations like the Pimas. Neel posited that genes that enable humans to store food as fat (the so-called thrifty genes) are beneficial when resources are scarce and unpredictable, but detrimental in times of constant abundance. This is a transition that the Pima Indians have recently made.

"People with a tendency to reduce the unsaturation of their membranes in times of famine could lower their metabolic rate and protect themselves against starvation," Storlien posits. "A fast metabolism is a very good thing if you're trying to maintain energy balance, but it is not a good thing in times of food shortage."*

Since teaming up with Hulbert and Else, Storlien has also found evidence that the composition of fatty acids strongly influences the binding of insulin to its receptor, in humans as well as rats, and that insulin sensitivity improves with increasing membrane unsaturation. But neither he nor anyone else has been able to produce what would be the most convincing support for this association between leaky membranes and syndrome X: a demonstrated improvement in insulin sensitivity among type 2 diabetics after the omega-3 fatty acids in their diets are increased. "It's driven most of us nuts," says Storlien. "It happens so easily in animals. Why doesn't it happen in humans?"

The reason may well be the same one that explains George and Mildred Burr's inability in the 1930s to prove that linoleic

---

*A very interesting implication of the work of Storlien, Hulbert, and Else, and one that has great relevance for the foods that people choose to eat, is that populations, when given the choice, will naturally drift toward foods with lesser amounts of omega-3s. Having a fast metabolism—the result, at least in part, of a diet rich in omega-3s—means having a greater requirement for food and a greater possibility, therefore, of going hungry. And being hungry is a far more unpleasant state than being overweight. This may be one reason why so many populations, the Inuit included, have adopted Western diets as soon as they have had the opportunity.

acid was essential to humans: people, especially obese people, carry huge fat reserves that buffer against change. "It would take years to turn over all of the fats on an obese person," says Storlien, "and I haven't been able to run my studies out that far. You don't get grants to do long-term intervention studies." That's why, he adds, the epidemiological data are so important. "The epidemiological data clearly show that fish intake is preventive against both heart disease and diabetes."

Not only has Storlien been unable to get funding for the kind of long-term study he would like to do, but he has also had difficulty publishing the results of some of the studies he *has* completed, including a one-year intervention in which a high omega-3 diet did result in an impressive improvement in insulin action as well as in a number of other lipid variables, triglycerides among them (improvements more marked than those achieved by the currently recommended high-carbohydrate diet). "This study was rejected by five journals," says Storlien. "Not because of the science, but because the reviewers said, 'You couldn't possibly get these effects from just changing the fatty acid profile of the diet.'"

Metabolism is remarkably complex, Storlien understands, and he is not trying to hang all his coats on one peg. Many independent factors contribute to diabetes and obesity (among them, activity and caloric intake). "But the pacemaker theory is a matter of a number of mechanisms coming together to push metabolism in a particular direction," he argues, "and it's time to test it with well-funded, long-term studies."

Storlien is frustrated that this work hasn't received more attention, but he knows that such recognition would require an acknowledgment that the effects of omega-3s and omega-6s are very different and that too great an intake of omega-6s can be harmful—a shift in message that very few governments have been willing to make. In 2000, Storlien took a research position with the pharmaceutical firm AstraZeneca in Sweden, but he continues to collaborate with Hulbert and Else. They have recently published a comprehensive paper on dietary fats and membrane function in *Biological Reviews*.

"We're missing the boat by not taking a more proactive stand on obesity," Storlien contends. "We should be taking the best thing we know about fatty acids and combining it with the best thing we know about proteins and carbohydrates."

"People are going to look back on this time—when we've flooded our food supply with omega-6s—like they do the Irish potato famine," says Hulbert, "as the unforeseen consequence of too heavy an emphasis on a single type of food." Artemis Simopoulos calls it "a human experiment of enormous proportions."

And what countries like the United States are also doing when they ignore the differences between the two families of essential fats is creating a climate in which the public doesn't believe anything the government has to say about fat, a climate in which faddish and dangerous diets thrive.

This brings me back to Atkins and the dietary madness with which this book began. For perhaps there is another reason why the Atkins diet and other low-carb diets are so popular in this day and age. These diets tend to be somewhat higher in protein than less restrictive regimes, and protein raises the body's metabolic rate by requiring us to get rid of excess nitrogen. This we can only do through the synthesis of urea, a process that requires a great deal of energy. Raising our metabolism in this way can have serious side effects (particularly stress on the kidney and liver that can lead to organ failure, as well as the wasting condition known to explorers as "rabbit starvation"). But could it be that the appeal of these diets is that they give us the kind of metabolic boost that we used to get through foods full of omega-3 fats? Could it be that they enable us to eat the quantity of food we were able to eat before the new foods in our diet slowed our metabolisms down? This is speculation, I know. But little else in my book is, and I hope that this short history of how scientists came to recognize that the Western world was deficient (insufficient, some prefer to say) in the most abundant fat on earth will help us to move forward and put omega-3s, the queen of fats, back into our foods. I hope that it will give us yet another reason for protecting our oceans and rivers, home to the most concentrated sources of these fats, and encourage us to develop new terrestrial sources of omega-3s that won't overtax those resources. Western food producers have succeeded in manufacturing remarkably cheap, pure, long-lasting foods that can satisfy all of a human's energy needs. But it is time we acknowledged that these foods do not meet all of our nutrition needs and that the health costs associated with these foods mean they are far from cheap.

"Good nutrition does not inevitably guarantee good health," observes Corinne Shear Wood in her book on human sickness and health. "Poor nutrition, however, always produces poor health." How great a bargain are our foods when the United States is spending 15 percent of its total economy, an average of $5,440 for each person, on health care? We are paying far more than is any other country—almost twice as much as Japan. This is not the first time that countries have created a nutritional deficiency with their agricultural and food-processing techniques (the epidemics of beriberi that followed the introduction of the practice of rice polishing come immediately to mind), and it probably won't be the last. But the problem needs to be recognized before it can be remedied. In the meantime, Simopoulos points out, "the advice to 'eat a balanced diet' makes no sense when our food has been stripped of one of its essential nutrients."

"We've changed our foods and we know how to change them back," says Norman Salem. Let's all hope so. Otherwise we will remain tethered to pharmaceutical and medical industries that can only fix this dietary problem badly—and at huge costs to society and the individual.

TWELVE

PUTTING OMEGA-3s BACK INTO *YOUR* FOOD SUPPLY

A good cook is half a physician.

ANDREW BOORDE, 1547

THE QUEEN OF FATS IS NOT A DIET OR A NUTRITION BOOK, NOR IS IT the last word in omega-3 recommendations or research, a field that expands greatly every year. But I would be remiss if I didn't give readers some advice on what fats they should be eating and how they can correct for the large amounts of linoleic acid in the American food supply. Though the government may dawdle over this issue, individual readers can take matters in their own hands by following some fairly simple and straightforward guidelines. These guidelines don't involve any calculations—calculations aren't necessary, and any food plan that does involve them is not one that free-foraging, free-ranging eaters, as most of us are, can adhere to over time. Besides, foods vary in their omega-3 content with season, location, and an animal's diet, so any figures I chose would be somewhat arbitrary. What I provide instead is a series of directions in which you can safely and confidently move.*

*Readers who would like more detailed shopping and cooking information, including recipes and a list of resources, should consult *The Omega Plan* by Artemis Simopoulos and Jo Robinson (New York: HarperCollins, 1998).

1. **EAT LOTS (AND LOTS) OF FRUITS AND VEGETABLES.** Green vegetables are full of alpha linolenic acid, the parent omega-3 fatty acid, and all fruits and vegetables contain antioxidants that protect fats against oxidation. To bulk up on alpha linolenic acid, you should eat the vegetables you enjoy—and lots of them. A number of seaweeds also have the ability to produce DHA or eicosapentaenoic acid and are an excellent addition to any diet.

2. **CONSUME OILS THAT HAVE A HEALTHY BALANCE OF OMEGA-3s AND OMEGA-6s.** Avoid oils in which linoleic acid greatly overshadows alpha linolenic acid, namely safflower, sunflower, corn, cottonseed, and peanut oils, and consume more flaxseed, walnut, canola, and soybean oils. It's even okay to eat small quantities of butter, which has large amounts of saturated fats and small amounts of polyunsaturated fats, but a wholesome ratio of omega-6s to omega-3s. Olive oil is another good alternative, though it too has only small amounts of alpha linolenic acid. But its amounts of linoleic acid are also small, and it is full of antioxidants and other beneficial compounds. Olive oil, of course, is one of the foundations (along with fish and vegetables) of the healthy, time-tested Mediterranean diet.

Though soybean oil is sometimes blamed for the current imbalance in our diets (probably because the rise in importance of soybeans as a crop has paralleled the increase of omega-6-rich linoleic acid in our food supply, and because most of the fat in the American diet—more than 75 percent—comes from this single source), soybean oil *can* be part of a wholesome diet. It should be used sparingly, and it shouldn't be hydrogenated or otherwise modified, as is much of the soybean oil in the United States. Most important, it shouldn't be your only source of omega-3s. Soybeans and soybean oil are part of the Japanese cuisine, and the Japanese, who also consume much more fish, vegetables, and seaweed than Western populations, have, as I've said, the longest life span and lowest rate of most diseases of any population on earth.

3. **EAT A WIDE VARIETY OF FISH.** Include lean fish such as cod, halibut, and trout in your diet as well as fatty fish such as salmon and mackerel. Because they live in water and require more flexibility in their membranes than do land animals, all fish are rich in omega-3 fatty acids. Fatty fish have more in their flesh because they store their excess fat in their bellies, not their livers, as do lean fish like cod. But all fish are a valuable source of these nutrients and should be appreciated as such. Eating a wide diversity of fish should help us to increase our omega-3 intake. It should also help to prevent overfishing and protect us against toxins that tend to accumulate in certain species.

4. **EAT OMEGA-3 ENRICHED EGGS.** Most grocery stores carry these—look for the words *omega-3s* or *DHA* on the carton. These eggs, laid by chickens that have been fed a diet rich in flaxseed, fish meal, and/or algae and other greens, provide one of the easiest ways of adding omega-3s to Western diets. They're easy to produce and less expensive than many other foods high in omega-3s. If the chickens are fed something other than fish meal, they're also free of the contaminants that can be found in fish.

Unfortunately, though, eggs are also the icon, or the poster child, of the anticholesterol campaign. They're the first food given up by people worried about serum cholesterol. Eggs have taken the greatest beating of any food in regard to cholesterol. But, says Ralph Holman, "if you get your omega-3 acids, they will take care of the cholesterol," a position supported by the work of William Connor at the Oregon Health and Science University in Portland and by studies that have found no association between egg consumption and either heart disease or serum cholesterol levels.* The Japanese, who consume some 340 eggs per person per year (100 or so more than most Americans), have a very low rate of heart disease.

By the way, omega-3s are concentrated in the yolks of eggs for the same reason that they're concentrated in breast milk and placental blood: to support the development—especially the brain development—of the next generation (in this case chickens instead of humans). An added benefit of enriching the diets of chickens with omega-3 fatty acids is that these chickens are healthier than others: they have better immune systems and fewer illnesses.

5. **TRY TO INCLUDE A SOURCE OF OMEGA-3s IN EVERY MEAL.** Doing so will enable alpha linolenic acid to exert its natural competitive edge over linoleic acid. The omega-3s can come from fish, greens, omega-3 enriched eggs, as well as cereals and breads containing whole and ground flaxseed. Other convenient sources of omega-3s are soy and other beans and some nuts: walnuts, notably, with lesser amounts in beechnuts,

---

* Because of these studies, the American Heart Association has eliminated earlier restrictions on the number of eggs that individuals are advised to consume. However, the AHA and governmental organizations still advocate a cholesterol intake of less than 300 mg/day—and in order to follow that recommendation, people have to limit their egg consumption to less than one daily. Or they have to forgo the yolk, the part of the egg richest in nutrients, including omega-3s. "People always tell me that they give their yolks to their dogs," says Donald McNamara, a researcher with the Egg Nutrition Center in Washington, D.C. "I tell them they have very healthy dogs."

Brazil nuts, and chestnuts. Most of these omega-3-rich ingredients can be added to salads, yogurts, cheeses, sauces, and so on. The nuts can be eaten as a snack (with or without raisins and chocolate chips). Homemade baked goods, such as breads, cookies, and cakes, can be a great source of omega-3s, especially if you add liberal amounts of walnuts, use omega-3-enriched eggs, and replace some of the butter with canola oil. Although omega-3s can also be taken in pill form (see below), like most nutrients, they are probably better absorbed from foods than pills.

6. **AVOID HYDROGENATED AND PARTIALLY HYDROGENATED OILS.** This step is important not only because of the reduced omega-3 content of these oils but also because of their concentrations of trans fats. Trans fats compete with cis fats for enzymes and positions in cell membranes, and they may have adverse effects of their own, though it is difficult to distinguish between the two. Avoiding these oils is fairly easy to do with foods bought in a grocery store, since producers are required to list them as ingredients on food labels. But the task is more difficult with foods consumed in restaurants. Short of asking a restaurant for a list of its ingredients (a step that takes the pleasure out of eating out), choose foods that are freshly prepared and pass on those that are packaged or fried. Many of the baked goods served in restaurants are also made with hydrogenated vegetable shortening instead of either butter or one of the healthy oils.

7. **CHOOSE FREE-RANGE CHICKEN, BEEF, BISON, AND PORK WHENEVER YOU CAN.** Because these animals have had to wander in search of food, they have more muscle and less fat than confined, grain-fed animals. And what fat they do have is much lower in saturates and much richer in polyunsaturates, espe-

cially omega-3s. When Michael Crawford compared the flesh of a wild Cape buffalo to a grain-fed steer, he found that the Cape buffalo had about one-tenth the amount of fat as the steer, but nearly six times the amount of omega-3 fatty acids. It's as if they were different foods altogether.

8. **CUT DOWN ON SATURATED FATS.** Though the association between heart disease and dietary cholesterol has not held up over the years, the one between heart disease and saturated fat has, and readers should cut down on these solid fats by choosing low-fat dairy products and lean cuts of meat. (The exception, of course, is the meat, or flesh, of fish; in that case, the fattier the better.) Saturated fats displace unsaturated fats in the diet and, in large amounts, they compete for enzymes and positions in cell membranes. They also increase the stickiness of platelets and the amount of low-density lipoproteins (LDLs) in the blood. The bottom line is that populations who decrease their intake of saturated fat and simultaneously increase their intake of omega-3s, as the Finns did in the 1970s and the northern Europeans did during the Second World War, successfully and dramatically lower their incidence of heart disease. Populations who decrease their intake of saturated fat and greatly increase their intake of omega-6s, the Israelis and Americans among them, see no such benefit.

9. **TAKE SPECIAL PRECAUTIONS IF YOU ARE PREGNANT OR A WOMAN OF REPRODUCTIVE AGE.** Follow the guidelines of the FDA and local agencies on fish consumption and look for fish that have tested negative for mercury and PCBs. Researchers are currently investigating whether the kind of mercury found in fish (methyl mercury cysteine) is less toxic than other forms; in the meantime, pregnant women should play it safe. Most important, they should supplement their diets with other

sources of omega-3s and keep their intake of omega-6s at healthy levels. The benefits will be enormous, not only for their babies but for themselves, since low maternal concentrations of DHA have been linked to an increased risk of postpartum depression. Omega-3 fatty acids have also been found to protect against preterm delivery and low birth weight. After giving birth, mothers should breast-feed whenever possible, since no formula on the market matches the breast milk of a well-nourished mother. If breast-feeding is not possible, parents should choose a formula supplemented with DHA and ARA (the formula companies' abbreviation for arachidonic acid) and not be fooled by formulas that say they support brain development yet lack these fatty acids.

10. USE SUPPLEMENTS CAREFULLY.   If you do take omega-3 supplements, avoid those that supply *all* the essential fatty acids, omega-6s and omega-3s. Omega-6s are essential, as we know, but we already have too many of them in our foods. We don't need to take any more. So avoid supplements (and foods) with phrases such as *high omega, complete omegas, complete EFA, ultimate omegas,* or *omega balance* in their names, as they will undoubtedly include oils rich in omega-6s. If you take fish oil, look for products that are of pharmaceutical grade or are molecularly distilled, thus ensuring that they will be free of metals and other toxins. Also, take fish oil rather than cod liver oil, as the latter contains significant amounts of vitamin A and can be harmful in excess.

As far as quantities go, researchers like Artemis Simopoulos recommend about 1 gram of DHA and eicosapentaenoic acid a day from food or supplements and 2 grams of alpha linolenic acid, but you'll need more alpha linolenic acid if you're a strict vegetarian or you don't eat fish regularly. Dosages as high as

3 to 8 grams of omega-3 fatty acids per day (10 to 27 grams of fish or flaxseed oil) lead to no adverse side effects and are generally well tolerated, though some people have problems with a "fishy" aftertaste (which can be avoided with lemon- or orange-flavored oils, such as those made by Nordic Naturals) and diarrhea (which can be avoided by lowering the dose). Needless to say, people with preexisting health problems should consult their physicians before beginning these supplements.

Keep your fish and flaxseed oils in a cool, dark place and throw out any oil that smells bad. (If it smells bad, it is bad. Taking oxidized oil is worse than taking no oil at all.) Individuals taking large amounts of flaxseed or flaxseed oil (including animals being raised with these oils in their diet) should also take vitamin B6, since flaxseeds contain a factor that interferes with this vitamin.

11. **MAINTAIN A HEALTHY WEIGHT BY GETTING THE EXERCISE AND CALORIES YOU NEED.** Excess calories and weight put a strain on the entire body and its systems, including its systems for storing and transporting fats.

Finally, don't go overboard with this or any diet. You need omega-6s in your diet, just not in the great quantities that most of us are currently getting. Saturated fats and monounsaturated fats are important for energy and the satiated feeling that helps us to leave the table after a meal, and the fat in any healthy diet will be mostly monounsaturated and saturated. Even trans fats cannot and should not be totally eliminated, since trans fats are found naturally in butter and other dairy products. Produced by the microbes in a cow's stomach, they constitute some 4 percent of the fats in butter. Balance is the key to this and every other aspect of life. By moving in the directions listed above, readers can be sure they will be changing the balance of fats in their tissues and confident that health benefits will follow. Omega-3s were displaced by the large amounts of linoleic acid in our diet. These eleven steps can restore the queen of fats to the throne.

THIRTEEN

THE PROOF IS IN THE PUDDING

I sometimes marvel how truth progresses, so difficult is it for one man to convince another, unless his mind is vacant.

CHARLES DARWIN, IN A LETTER TO ALFRED RUSSEL WALLACE, 1868

AS FRUSTRATED AS SCIENTISTS SUCH AS RALPH HOLMAN AND William Lands are with the slow pace of acceptance of the importance of omega-3s, it is just a matter of time, they know, until the work catches on. Let me put it this way: It is just a matter of time until a person's omega-3 status will replace serum cholesterol, LDL to HDL ratio, and even C-reactive protein, the newest, hottest risk factor (and one that is highly correlated with omega-3 status), to assess that person's risk for sudden cardiac death and other diseases. It is just a matter of time until patients who are at risk will be advised to change the fats in their diet instead of taking statins and other costly medications. Statins, by the way, have been found to help patients with high cholesterol not by blocking cholesterol synthesis (which they do) but by reducing inflammation and the tendency toward clot formation. This, of course, is the effect that a high omega-3 diet would have—without any of the statins' adverse side reactions.

Patients will scratch their heads and wonder what happened to all of those earlier medicines, recommendations, risk factors, and tests, and some may find the answer in this book. But the change is inevitable. The current tests will go the way of all not-so-revealing medical assays, including the elaborate urine tests of the fifteenth century and the phrenology maps of the early nineteenth century. Recommendations to reduce dietary cholesterol and block the synthesis of cholesterol (a necessary component of brain function) will one day seem as quaint and outdated as bloodletting.

How can I, or any of these researchers, be so certain, you might ask?

The best reason is the very thing that has been missing in all the decades that we have been pursuing serum cholesterol as the quarry in our fight against heart disease: a clear, biologically plausible mechanism linking eicosapentaenoic acid and DHAs (a dearth of them, of course) to an increased risk for heart disease. Mechanisms, I should say, since there are more than one. An increased susceptibility to abnormal and lethal heart rhythms leads the list, followed closely by an increased tendency toward inflammation and thrombosis. To make a short narrative out of what we know about omega-3s and heart disease: a heart that is deficient in these fats beats less vigorously, and the arteries leading out of it tend to silt up with fats, especially those of the solid variety. Those arteries are also deficient in omega-3s, and the silting, even the normal wear and tear of blood flow, produces inflammatory eicosanoids and inflammatory proteins like C-reactive protein, ineffective attempts to patch the inflamed tissues with cholesterol, and oxidation of the cholesterol and other fats, as well as an increase in blood pressure and clotting tendency, which put ever more stress on this poorly nourished heart. In some people, this unfortunate cascade of events leads to thrombosis; in others, arrhythmia.

Our certainty is also based on the epidemiological data linking omega-3 consumption to a population's risk of heart disease, which are consistent both between and within populations. And that is much more than you can say for the epidemiological data linking heart disease and either cholesterol or fat consumption, Ancel Keys's 1953 chart notwithstanding. The latter is not consistent for reasons that scientists who know to distinguish between *all* the different families of fats now understand—that is, the kind of fat that a population consumes matters much more than the quantity.

Finally, there are the many prospective and intervention studies showing how omega-3 status changes the outlook for heart disease. In one intervention trial with patients who had already suffered one heart attack, 11,000 subjects were given either one capsule of DHA and eicosapentaenoic acid daily (850 milligrams) or the usual care, and then followed for three and a half years. In the patients who took the supplement, the risk of sudden death from a heart attack was reduced by 45 percent; the risk for death from any cause, by 20 percent.

In a prospective study within the Physicians' Health Study, which began in 1982 and is expected to end in 2007, 14,916 healthy male physicians were followed for a period of seventeen years. During that time, 94 of them experienced sudden cardiac death. Investigators compared the amount of omega-3s in the blood of all the subjects and concluded that the risk for sudden cardiac death was reduced by 90 percent in those whose levels were highest.

In another recent analysis, of 222,000 individuals who were being followed for coronary heart disease for an average of twelve years (in thirteen different cohorts or groups), those people who consumed just one meal of fish per week had a 15 percent reduction in risk, as compared with those who consumed less than one meal of fish per month. Those people who consumed five or more meals of fish per week, the highest category of fish consumption, showed a 40 percent reduction in risk.

These are just three of the more than 4,500 studies that have explored the effects of omega-3 fatty acids on human health since Dyerberg and Bang's first trips to Greenland in the 1970s, and by and large, the message of these studies is consistent and clear. We ignore it at our peril and at the price of continued poor health.

What aren't as clear, at this point, are all the diseases in which omega-3s play a part; all the mechanisms by which omega-3s act; and all the factors—aging, smoking, pregnancy, genetic variation, alcohol and antioxidant intake, and so on—that affect an individual's omega-3 status. Also in question is the best measurement of an individual's omega-3 status to determine risk of heart disease and other illnesses.

Is it, as the physician Clemens von Schacky and William S. Harris (a colleague of William Connor's) have recently suggested, the percentage of DHA and eicosapentaenoic acid in the fatty acids of red blood cell membranes, a percentage that has been shown to be highly correlated with cardiac membrane omega-3 fatty acid levels and that they have dubbed the *omega-3 index?*

Or is it what researchers are calling the *inflammatory index*, the ratio of arachidonic acid to eicosapentaenoic acid in red blood cells?

Or the widely used omega-6 to omega-3 ratio, a ratio that includes all the omega-6s in red blood cells in the numerator and all the omega-3s in the denominator?

Or the index recommended by William Lands, the amount of omega-3 HUFAs as a percentage of total HUFAs in any tissue, including a drop of whole blood? (A HUFA, remember, is a highly unsaturated fatty acid, defined as a fatty acid with twenty or more carbons and three or more double bonds.)

All of these indices have something to recommend them as markers of omega-3 status, and time will tell which are the most useful for predicting who is at risk for heart disease, cancer, depression, and all the other maladies that are being associated with an insufficiency of omega-3s. There is much still to be learned, but that shouldn't keep us from benefiting immediately from the predictive power of omega-3s.

To date, only a few physicians are requesting fatty acid tests for their patients, but individuals who would like to know whether the fats in their bodies put them in the company of the Eskimos or the Americans, the Japanese or the Israelis, in terms of their risk of disease can have their blood tested by one of several companies. If you live in a state that permits direct testing by consumers, you can request a test kit from OmegaMetrix in Kansas City, Missouri (1–866–677–4900; www.omegametrix.com), and follow the directions for having your blood tested. No matter where you live, you can request a test from Your Future Health in Tavares, Florida (1–877–468–6934; www.yourfuturehealth.com); ask your physician to request a test from Nutrasource Diagnostics in Guelph, Ontario (call William Rowe, the president of the company, at 1–519–824–4120, ext. 58817); or contact Doug Bibus, a colleague of Ralph Holman's, at bibus@omega3health.com. These tests are fairly expensive, totaling $115 at OmegaMetrix and $285 at Your Future Health, but their cost may come down as they are used more widely. (Readers should be wary of the tendency at some of these companies to overinterpret results.)

Once you switch to a high omega-3, low omega-6 diet, you can expect to see significant changes in your blood almost immediately, paralleled by a rapid improvement in heart function and mood, as experienced by Dale Jarvis and others who have supplemented their diets with large amounts of omega-3s. Other benefits, such as a speedier metabolic rate, will take much longer (two to three years, depending on how much adipose tissue you carry) but are worth waiting for.

The one thing readers shouldn't expect is any surprises. If you are eating a typical fast-food diet, your cells will be full of omega-6s. If you are avoiding processed foods and partially hydrogenated fats and are eating a lot of greens and fish, your cells will have a good balance of omega-3s and omega-6s. In the matter of fats, we truly are what we eat and what we eat truly matters.

TIME LINE

SOME IMPORTANT EVENTS IN THE LONG, UNFINISHED TALE OF OMEGA-3 RESEARCH

1792—Jean Senebier, a Swiss clergyman and scientist, observes that exposure to air causes oils to go white, lose their fluidity, and in time go rancid. Further investigation convinces him that rancidity involves oxidation.

1814—Michel Eugène Chevreul, a French scientist, shows that hog's lard consists of two distinct oily bodies. One is a solid at room temperature and the other, a liquid.

1887 A fatty acid with three double bonds is described. It is called linolenic acid and first found in hempseed oil.

1897—The French chemist Paul Sabatier describes the hardening (hydrogenation) of fats in the presence of a metallic catalyst, a discovery for which he wins a Nobel Prize in 1912.

1900—V. D. Anderson in Cleveland, Ohio, manufactures the first continuous screw press—known as the "expeller"—for extracting oil from oil seeds. The expeller is much more efficient than earlier hydraulic presses, but it still leaves much of the oil in the meal and much room, therefore, for improvement.

1903—The German chemist Wilhelm Norman takes out a patent for the "conversion of unsaturated fatty acids . . . into saturated compounds" by hydrogenation.

1911—Procter and Gamble introduce Crisco, a solid vegetable fat made by hydrogenating cottonseed oil, thus providing a lost-cost, vegetable-derived alternative to butter and lard.

—The first commercial quantities of soybeans are imported into America from Manchuria and crushed for oil.

1929—George and Mildred Burr discover that certain fats are essential for the growth and survival of rats, causing scientists to rethink the idea that fats are necessary only as a source of calories and fat-soluble vitamins.

1930—Gynecologists working with artificial insemination report that extracts of seminal fluid cause uterine tissue to contract, an observation that leads to the discovery of the important cell messengers called *prostaglandins*.

1931—The Burrs identify the essential factor in fats required by rats: the unsaturated fat linoleic acid. Later they find that either linolenic acid or archidonic acid can replace linoleic acid.

—Henry Ford plants 500 acres in Dearborn, Michigan, in soybeans. Before the Second World War, the United States imports about 40 percent of its edible oils and fats. After the war, and after soybean production takes off, the country is able to export edible oils.

1934—Archer Daniels Midland Company opens the first continuous countercurrent solvent extraction plant in the United States, using hexane as the solvent and a 100-tons-per-day Hildebrandt extractor from Germany. By the late 1940s, much of the oil seed–crushing industry moves from screw presses to far more efficient solvent extraction.

1938—The Burrs are unable to prove that linoleic acid is essential for humans and the question remains unresolved until the 1960s.

1950—Ralph Holman and a graduate student discover that linoleic acid is the precursor of arachidonic acid and that alpha linolenic acid is the precursor of DHA and eicosapentaenoic acid.

1951—Two English scientists, A. J. P. Martin and A. J. James, perfect the first gas-liquid chromatograph, a powerful analytical and purification tool that enables scientists to separate the many different fatty acids in tissues and foods; for this work, they shared the Nobel Prize in 1952.

—Herbert Dutton proves that linolenic acid is the cause of the off flavors and odors in soybean oil, leading to the expanded use of partial or selective hydrogenation to eliminate this fat.

1953—Ancel Keys publishes a chart that seems to show that the incidence of heart disease is directly correlated with the total fat intake of a population.

1955—Trans fatty acids are found to be naturally present in ruminants but not nonruminants.

1957—Sune Bergström isolates the first prostaglandins.

1960—Holman describes the presence of high amounts of Mead's acid (20:3ω9) in animals deprived of essential fatty acids.

1962—Holman's mother dies of a deficiency of linoleic acid, one of several cases leading to the recognition that linoleic acid, the parent omega-6 fat, is essential for humans.

1964—Holman proposes a new system for naming the different families of unsaturated fatty acids, the omega system, and hypothesizes that the different families compete for the same elongation and desaturation enzymes.

—Bergström and David van Dorp demonstrate that prostaglandins are made from twenty-carbon fatty acids, such as arachidonic and eicosapentaenoic acid.

1967—Trout raised with corn oil as the only fat in their diet develop a shock syndrome and suffer a high mortality. Trout are the first animal to be recognized as requiring omega-3 fatty acids.

1968—Michael Crawford presents evidence that the fats of domestic animals are much more saturated than the fats of wild animals.

1972—Hans Olaf Bang and Jørn Dyerberg report that compared to Danes, Greenland Eskimos have lower levels of heart disease—and of serum cholesterol and triglycerides, despite a diet rich in fat and blubber.

—Crawford presents the first evidence that DHA is important to brain function.

1973—William Lands reports that prostaglandins made from omega-3 fatty acids are much less inflammatory than those made from omega-6 fatty acids, a finding that leads to the use of fish oil in treating patients with arthritis, ulcerative colitis, Crohn's disease, dysmenorrhea, and other inflammatory disorders.

1975—Robert Anderson identifies DHA as a key part of the eye's photoreceptor.

1977—A report by the World Health Organization concludes that infant formulas should match the milk from well-nourished mothers with respect both to parent and long-chain fatty acids and to the balance of the omega-6 and omega-3 families.

1978—Bang, Dyerberg, and John Vane suggest that eicosapentaenoic acid, an omega-3 fat, plays a role in the prevention of thrombosis and atherosclerosis.

—Six-year-old Shawna Strobel is shot in the stomach by her caretaker's husband.

1982—Ralph Holman and his colleagues report that the neurological symptoms of Shawna Strobel, who has been living on a total parenteral nutrition formula ever since her gunshot wound, are caused by a deficiency of omega-3 fatty acids. Omega-3s come to be recognized as essential for humans (as well as trout), but it's thought to be almost impossible to make someone deficient in this widespread nutrient.

—Bergström, Bengt Samuelsson, and Vane receive the Nobel Prize for their discoveries relating to prostaglandins.

1985—Scientists begin linking an imbalance of omega-6s and omega-3s to numerous diseases, raising questions about the food supply of Western countries.

1986—Artemis Simopoulos reports that there are more omega-3 fatty acids in leaves than in seeds—and in the leaves of wild plants like purslane than in cultivated plants.

1987—Leonard Storlien finds that fish oil prevents insulin resistance and obesity in rats.

1989—The DART (Diet and Reinfarction Trial) and GISSI (Gruppo Italiano per lo Studio della Sopravvivenza nell'Infarto miocardico) trials reveal the benefits of omega-3 fatty acids in preventing death from myocardial infarction. Similar findings—that is, that fish consumption as low as 35 grams per day, or about one serving a week, significantly reduces the risk of myocardial infarction—are later reported by the Chicago Western Electric, MRFIT (Multiple Risk Factor Intervention Trial), and Honolulu Heart Program studies.

—Dennis Hoffman is the first of a number of investigators to find significant differences in the visual and mental acuity of infants raised on formulas with and without omega-3 fatty acids.

1995—Alexander Leaf reports that omega-3 fatty acids also prevent arrhythmia and sudden cardiac death.

1999—Joe Hibbeln and Andrew Stoll independently report that there is an inverse correlation between omega-3 consumption and the incidence of depression and that fish oil reduces episodes of mania and depression in patients with bipolar disorder.

—Tony Hulbert and Paul Else publish data indicating that the degree of unsaturation of an animal's membranes, a function, in part, of the dietary intake of omega-3s and omega-6s, is the pacemaker of that animal's metabolism. This discovery creates a new way of looking at the role that greens and seeds play in human health and a framework on which to hang all the other findings about omega-3s.

GLOSSARY

ACYLTRANSFERASES—The enzymes responsible for assembling phospholipids.

ALPHA LINOLENIC ACID (ALA)—An eighteen-carbon fatty acid that is the parent of the essential omega-3 family of fats; plants use it in photosynthesis and in the formation of cell messengers. It is therefore found mostly in green leaves and is the most abundant fat on the planet. Only plants can turn linoleic acid into alpha linolenic acid (by adding a double bond), but most animals, including humans, can turn alpha linolenic acid into the longer and more desaturated eicosapentaenoic acid and DHA. See linoleic acid.

ANTIOXIDANTS—Naturally occurring compounds that neutralize free radicals (see below) before they can cause cell damage.

ARACHIDONIC ACID (abbreviated AA, or sometimes ARA)—A twenty-carbon omega-6 fatty acid, found throughout the body, that is the source of the most potent and inflammatory eicosanoids. Most animals, including humans, can make AA from linoleic acid. It can also be consumed ready-made; foods particularly rich in AA are meats and other animal products.

ARRHYTHMIA—A disturbance in the coordinated rhythmic contraction of the heart muscle.

CANOLA OIL—A vegetable oil developed in Canada during the late 1960s and early 1970s and introduced into the United States in 1985. Canola oil is extracted from a hybrid form of rapeseed that is very low in erucic acid, a twenty-two-carbon monounsaturated fatty acid that had been found to cause fatty deposits in the hearts of test animals. Most rapeseed contains more than 30 percent erucic acid, but the kind used to make canola oil has only 0.3 to 1.2 percent. Canola oil gets its name from a melding of *Canada* and *oil*; it is also called LEAR (low erucic acid rapeseed) oil. It is known for having a significant alpha linolenic acid content (and for being low in saturates and high in monounsaturates), but none of these attributes is fixed; and, as is also true of soy and other oil seeds, new varieties of canola are being developed all the time.

CHLOROPLASTS—Specialized structures within plant cells that contain stacks and stacks of membranes in which the many proteins involved in photosynthesis are embedded. The membrane, called the *thylacoid membrane*, is the most abundant thing on the planet. Thus its major fat, alpha linolenic acid, is the most abundant fat. Shown below is an electromicrograph of one of the many chloroplasts in a cell from the leaf of a tobacco plant *(Nicotiana tobacum)*, courtesy of Richard McAvoy and Mariya Khodakovskaya.

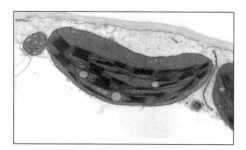

CIS CONFORMATION—A double bond in which the two hydrogens are on the same side, thus forming a kink or bend in the molecule that dramatically lowers its melting point (the temperature at which it goes from being a solid to a liquid). In most naturally occurring fats, all the double bonds are in the cis conformation.

$$-C=C-$$
$$\ \ |\ \ |$$
$$\ \ H\ H$$

DESATURASES—Enzymes that introduce double bonds into specific sites on fatty acids. Only plants have the delta-12 and the delta-15 desaturases that can turn oleic acid into linoleic acid and linoleic acid into alpha linolenic acid (by adding double bonds before the twelfth and fifteenth carbons—the sixth and the third, if you count backward). Animals (and some plants) have the delta-5, delta-6, and delta-9 desaturases.

DESATURATION—The removal of hydrogen atoms to create a double bond between two carbons. See unsaturated bonds.

DOCOSAHEXAENOIC ACID (DHA)—A twenty-two-carbon omega-3 fatty acid that is found in the largest amounts in a body's most active tissues. the brain, eyes, and heart. With twenty-two carbons and six double bonds, DHA is the longest, most unsaturated fatty acid in most living things. Most animals, including humans, can make DHA from alpha linolenic acid and eicosapentaenoic acid, or it can be consumed already-made. Foods that are rich in DHA include brains and fish, fish oils, and other seafoods, including some seaweeds.

DOUBLE BOND—A chemical bond in which two pairs (rather than a single pair) of electrons are shared between two atoms. When double bonds form between carbon atoms, those carbons do not share as many electrons with hydrogen atoms and the bond is said to be unsaturated.

EICOSANOIDS—A group of cell messengers that includes all the prostaglandins, thromboxanes, and leukotrienes (see below). Eicosanoids are formed from twenty-carbon highly unsaturated fatty acids (HUFAs) by either the cyclooxygenase (COX) or lipoxygenase (LOX) enzymes; they affect blood pressure, blood clotting, immune function, allergic response, reproduction, uterine muscle contraction, gastric secretion, and other important processes.

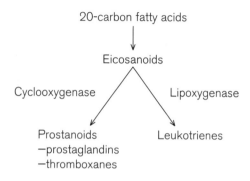

EICOSAPENTAENOIC ACID (EPA)—A twenty-carbon omega-3 fatty acid that is the source of the least inflammatory eicosanoids. Most animals, including humans, can make EPA from alpha linolenic acid, or it can be consumed already-made. Foods rich in EPA include fish, fish oils, and other seafoods.

ELONGASES—Enzymes that elongate fatty acids. Because they always add two carbons at a time, fatty acids always have an even number of carbons.

ESSENTIAL FATTY ACIDS—The fatty acids that animals cannot make themselves but require for health, including alpha linolenic acid and linoleic acid. AA, EPA, and DHA are also essential for health; but since animals can make them out of alpha linolenic acid and linoleic acid, these longer fatty acids are sometimes called *conditionally* essential.

FATS—A form of fatty acids used in storage and transport. Insoluble in water, they are made by combining three fatty acids and one molecule of glycerol. Fats can be either solids or liquids, depending on whether the fatty acids they are made from are mostly saturated or unsaturated. The fats in butter, lard, and coconut oil have many saturated fatty acids. The fats in vegetable and fish oil have many unsaturated fatty acids. *See* triglycerides.

FATTY ACID—A string of carbons and hydrogens attached to a weak carboxylic acid. The acidic part of a fatty acid is lost when it combines with glycerol and two other fatty acids to make a triglyceride or molecule of fat. The fatty acids in living tissues are generally sixteen to twenty-two carbons long and have zero to six double bonds. Palmitic acid, an important component of palm oil and animal fats, is sixteen carbons long and fully saturated. Stearic, oleic, linoleic, and alpha linolenic acid are all eighteen carbons long and have zero, one, two, and three double bonds, respectively. Oleic acid, the main fatty acid in olive oil, is also the most abundant fat in animal tissues. Alpha linolenic acid is the most abundant fatty acid in plant tissues (and, therefore, the world), and DHA is the longest and most desaturated fatty acid in most animal tissues.

FREE RADICALS—Highly reactive molecules that can alter or destroy neighboring molecules and are controlled by antioxidants. Free radical reactions in tissues can cause cancer and atherosclerosis; reactions in foods can damage their odor, taste, and color.

GAS-LIQUID CHROMATOGRAPHY—A method for separating and analyzing the different fatty acids in a tissue or fat. It relies on the differential mobility of those molecules in a support medium.

HIGHLY UNSATURATED FATTY ACIDS (HUFAs)—Fatty acids that contain three or more double bonds and are at least twenty carbons long. The most important HUFAs in the body are AA, DGLA (dihomo-gamma-linolenic acid), EPA, and DHA. Animals make Mead's acid, a HUFA derived from oleic acid, only when they are deficient in essential fats.

HYDROGENATION—The chemical conversion of polyunsaturated vegetable or fish oils into solid (saturated) fats by the addition of hydrogen to all the double bonds. This process, invented at the turn of the twentieth century, requires the presence of a metal catalyst.

INFLAMMATION—A local response to stimuli that often involves redness, heat, pain, swelling, and loss of normal tissue function due to a release of inflammatory eicosanoids and other mediators.

LEUKOTRIENES—A kind of eicosanoid formed from the action of a lipoxygenase (LOX) enzyme on twenty-carbon highly unsaturated fatty acids. *See* eicosanoids.

LINOLEIC ACID—An eighteen-carbon fatty acid with two double bonds that is the parent of the essential omega-6 family of fatty acids. Plants store most of the fat in their seeds as linoleic acid, which they convert to alpha linolenic acid upon germination. As the use of seed oils has increased in the United States and other Western countries, linoleic acid has become much more prevalent in diets than alpha linolenic acid.

LINOLENIC ACID—Any of several fatty acids with three double bonds. Alpha linolenic acid, the parent omega-3 fatty acid, is the most prevalent form of linolenic acid, but several omega-6 forms also exist. *See* alpha linolenic acid.

LIPID—A compound that is not very soluble in water because of its many carbon atoms. The most abundant lipid in living tissues is fat or triglycerides; other important lipids are cholesterol and phospholipids.

LIPOPROTEIN—An assembly of lipids and proteins used by living tissues. Lipoproteins in the blood carry fats around the body. The nonpolar fats and cholesterol are in the middle of these assemblies, shielded from the water-based blood, and the proteins and polar lipids (including the phospholipids) are on the outside. Interactions of these proteins with proteins on the surfaces of cells and with enzymes in the blood determine whether triglycerides and cholesterol will be added to or removed from the lipoprotein. High-density lipoproteins collect cholesterol from the body's tissues and bring it back to the liver. Low-density lipoproteins carry cholesterol from the liver to the cells of the body.

MEAD'S ACID—*See* highly unsaturated fatty acids.

MEMBRANES—The millionth-of-a-centimeter-thick envelopes that enclose our cells and the components within them. Membranes control traffic in and out of cells; proteins embedded in them conduct most of a cell's business. The backbone of every membrane is a bilayer of phospholipids: the phosphorus groups are on the outside and the fatty tails are buried in the middle. The ability of phospholipids to form bilayers is built into their molecular structure. Below is a representation of a section of the highly unsaturated membrane of the rod cells of the eye (adapted from D. C. Mitchell, K. Gawrisch, B. J. Litman, and N. Salem, Jr., et al., "Why Is Docosahexaenoic Acid Essential for Nervous System Function?" *Biochemical Society Transactions* 26 [1998]: 368).

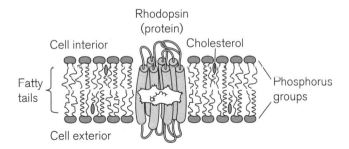

OLEIC ACID—An eighteen-carbon fatty acid with one double bond. Oleic acid is abundant in olive oil and can be formed by all living things—animals as well as plants. Its double bond is before the ninth-to-last carbon, and it is therefore known as an omega-9.

OMEGA-3s—A family of polyunsaturated fatty acids that originate in the green leaves of plants and share a double bond before the third to the last of their carbons. Omega-3s weren't known to be essential until the 1980s; by that time, a variety of food-processing techniques had all but eliminated them from many foods. By classical definition, a true omega-3 deficiency is rare, but a relative insufficiency, whose effects may approach those of a true deficiency, is now considered prevalent.

OMEGA-6s—A family of polyunsaturated fatty acids that share a double bond before the sixth-to-last carbon and compete with omega-3s for enzymes and positions in cell membranes. A high omega-6 to omega-3 ratio has been linked to many human diseases.

OMEGA-9s—A family of unsaturated family acids that originate with oleic acid and share a double bond before the ninth-to-last carbon.

OXIDATION—The addition of oxygen to a chemical structure. In oils, oxidation causes rancidity.

PACEMAKER THEORY—The theory (also called the *leaky membrane hypothesis*) that an animal's metabolic rate is determined by the number and type of unsaturated fatty acids in its cell membranes.

PARTIAL HYDROGENATION—A chemical process for adding hydrogen atoms to only some of the double bonds in polyunsaturated fatty acids, leaving others intact or turning them into trans bonds. Also known as *selective hydrogenation*, partial hydrogenation eliminates the alpha linolenic acid in an oil but leaves most of the linoleic acid.

PHOSPHOLIPASES—The enzymes that release fatty acids from membranes so that they can be turned into eicosanoids.

PHOSPHOLIPIDS—A major component of cell membranes. Phospholipids resemble triglycerides except that a polar phosphate group has replaced one of the three hydrocarbons, thereby giving phospholipids a water-insoluble *and* a water-soluble part and leading to the spontaneous formation of the bilayers that make up membranes.

PLATELETS—A specialized type of blood cell that adheres to blood vessel walls and can aggregate to form a clot, or thrombus.

POLYUNSATURATED FATTY ACIDS (PUFAs)—Fatty acids containing at least two double bonds.

PROSTACYCLIN—A type of prostaglandin produced by the endothelial cells of blood vessels that counteracts the tendency of blood to form clots.

PROSTAGLANDIN—A type of eicosanoid that is formed following the action of a cyclooxygenase (COX) enzyme on twenty-carbon highly unsaturated fatty acids.

SATURATED FATTY ACIDS—A fatty acid in which all the bonds between the carbons have the full complement of hydrogens—i.e., there are no double bonds.

THROMBOXANE—An eicosanoid derived from a prostaglandin intermediate that causes the aggregation of platelets and the contraction of muscles.

TRANS CONFORMATION—A double bond in which the two hydrogens are on the opposite sides of the molecule. Trans bonds force hydrocarbons into a more linear, zigzag conformation and dramatically raise the temperature at which they go from being a solid to a liquid. Trans fats are formed during the partial hydrogenation of fats. They are also formed by bacteria in the stomachs of ruminants and are naturally present in small amounts in butter and other dairy products.

$$\begin{array}{c} H \\ | \\ -C\!=\!C- \\ | \\ H \end{array}$$

TRIGLYCERIDES—A technical name for fats and the predominant component of food fats and oils. Triglycerides with two or more saturated fatty acids produce fats that are solid at room temperature, such as butter, lard, and coconut oil. Triglycerides with two or more unsaturated fatty acids produce fats that are liquid at room temperature, such as vegetable and fish oils. Shown below is a triglyceride made up of three saturated fatty acids.

UNSATURATED BOND—A double bond between two carbon atoms in a carbon compound. Since these carbons do not have the full complement of hydrogens, the bond is said to be *unsaturated*.

NOTES

P. 5   *DHA is a quick-change artist*   Readers who know that the cis double bonds in polyunsaturated fatty acids are more rigid and have significantly fewer degrees of freedom than the single bonds in saturated fatty acids, the result of repulsive forces between the hydrogen atoms on double-bonded carbons, may find the notion of DHA as a quick-change artist confusing. But a new and more accurate understanding of DHA has emerged very recently from studies using nuclear magnetic resonance and other techniques. To explain this flexibility, Klaus Gawrisch at the National Institute of Health's Laboratory of Membrane Biochemistry and Biophysics points to the extremely low potential barriers to rotation about the carbon-carbon bonds *between* the double bonds: these permit DHA, and other polyunsaturated fatty acids, to rapidly change conformation without expending significant energy. William Stillwell and Stephen R. Wassall discuss the unusual properties of DHA in "Docosahexaenoic Acid: Membrane Properties of a Unique Fatty Acid," *Chemistry and Physics of Lipids* 126 (2003): 1–27; see also D.C. Mitchell, K. Gawrisch, B.J. Litman, and N. Salem, Jr., "Why Is Docosahexaenoic Acid Essential for Nervous System Function?" *Biochemical Society Transactions* 26 (1998): 365–70.

P. 7   *And this rarity*   I will not attempt to cite the many thousands of studies linking deficiency in omega-3s to a long and growing list of illnesses. For an overview of the field and a more complete list of references, see Andrew Stoll, *The Omega Connection* (New York: Simon and Schuster, 2001); William Lands, *Fish and Human Health* (Orlando, FL: Academic Press, 1986); or Artemis Simopoulos and Jo Robinson, *The Omega Plan* (New York: HarperCollins, 1998). Other excellent resources are William E. Connor's "Importance of n-3 Fatty Acids in Health and Disease," *American Journal of Clinical Nutrition* 71 (2000): 171S–175S, and the Power-Pak program for pharmacists, physicians, nurses, and dieticians written by Doug Bibus and released August 1, 2001: *Omega-3s: Implications in Human Health and Disease* (for availability, contact Power-Pak at www.powerpak.com).

Also, I assert that there is a connection between an insufficiency of omega-3s and certain kinds of cancers even though a RAND Corporation study published in January 2006 in the *Journal of the American Medical Association* found no significant association between omega-3s and the incidence of any cancers. This study, like so many attempting to understand the role of specific fats in health and disease, failed to take into account the competitive interactions between different fats and to understand that no fat can be examined in a vacuum. It is for this reason that epidemiological studies and animal studies, many of which do show striking associations between a high percentage of omega-3s in the diet and low incidences of certain cancers, are so important. Epidemiological findings are a reflection of total dietary intake over long periods of time; the diets of experimental animals can be precisely controlled. Experimental studies are also revealing the actual mechanisms whereby omega-3 fatty acids reduce cancer growth, some of which are discussed in later chapters. (Catherine H. MacLean et al., "Effects of Omega-3 Fatty Acids on Cancer Risk," *Journal of the American Medical Association* 295 [2006].)

P. 9   *But it's time we learned that certain fats*   A. J. Hulbert, N. Turner, L.H. Storlien, and P. L. Else, "Dietary Fats and Membrane

Function: Implications for Metabolism and Disease," *Biological Reviews* 80 (2005): 155–69.

P. 10   *The new strains*   Soybeans typically produce oil with about 7 percent alpha linolenic acid. A new variety created by researchers at Iowa State University produces oil with only 1 percent. A university spokesperson, while boasting that this oil, which was developed through conventional hybridization, will help reduce the amount of trans fats in the food supply, does not mention that it will also reduce the amount of omega-3s (Walter Fehr, "New Soybean Oil Eliminates Need for Hydrogenation and Cuts Trans Fats," *Ag Decision Maker Newsletter*, November 2003,www.extension.iastate.edu/agdm/articles/others/FehrNov03 .htm [accessed January 7, 2005]). Varieties of rapeseed used to produce canola oil generally have 8 to 10 percent alpha linolenic acid, but one new variety has only 3 percent (R. K. Downey, "Canola: A Quality Brassica Oilseed," in *Advances in New Crops: Proceedings of the First National Symposium NEW CROPS, Research, Development, Economics, Indianapolis, Indiana, October 23–26, 1988*, ed. Jules Janick and James E. Simon [Portland, OR: Timber Press, 1990], 211–17). See also "Researchers Report Gains in Hunt for Low-Linolenic Soybeans," *Journal of the American Oil Chemists Society* 59 (1982): 882A–884A.

P. 11   *At a time when more than 70 percent*   William J. Broad and Andrew C. Revkin, "Has the Sea Given Up Its Bounty?" *Science Times*, July 29, 2003, F1.

P. 11   *They collected data*   P. M. Kris-Etherton et al., "Polyunsaturated Fatty Acids in the Food Chain in the United States," *American Journal of Clinical Nutrition* 71 (2000): 179S–188S.

P. 12   *The second-highest concentration of DHA*   The high concentration of DHA in sperm raises the question of whether reports of a decline in human sperm density (i.e., millions of sperm per milliliter semen) since the 1950s are linked to changes in our food supply. One paper has linked DHA levels to sperm motility (N. M. Gulaya et al., "Phospholipid Composition of Human Sperm and Seminal Plasma in Relation to

Sperm Fertility," *Archives of Andrology* 46 [2001]: 169–75), but this important issue deserves more study.

The data on hummingbirds and rattlesnakes come from biologists at Cornell University who were interested in testing the hypothesis of the Australian researchers Tony Hulbert and Paul Else, cited above, and used hummingbirds that they found, dead, at feeders and other places; see Juan P. Infante, Ryan C. Kirwan, and J. Thomas Brenna, "High Levels of Docosahexaenoic Acid (22:6n-3)-Containing Phospholipids in High-Frequency Contraction Muscles of Hummingbirds and Rattlesnakes," *Comparative Biochemistry and Physiology*, Part B, 130 (2001): 291–98. The finding on marmots comes from Vanessa L. Hill and Gregory L. Florant, "The Effect of a Linseed Oil Diet on Hibernation in Yellow-Bellied Marmots *(Marmota flaviventris)*," *Physiology and Behavior* 68 (2000): 431–37, and that on the athletes from Agneta Andersson, Anders Sjödin, Anu Hedman, Roger Olsson, and Bengt Vessby, "Fatty Acid Profile of Skeletal Muscle Phospholipids in Trained and Untrained Young Men," *American Journal of Physiological Endocrinology and Metabolism* 279 (2000): E744–51. The trained and untrained young men in this study ate the same diet, by the way, so the difference in DHA is the result of some sort of preference or selectivity of trained muscle fibers for this long and very active fatty acid. The study of the Pima Indians is by David P. Pan, Stephen Lilloja, Michael R. Milner, Amandia D. Kriketos, Louise A. Baur, Clifton Bogardus, and L. H. Storlien, "Skeletal Muscle Membrane Lipid Composition Is Related to Adiposity and Insulin Action," *Journal of Clinical Investigation* 96 (1995): 2802–8.

TWO. A TRIP TO GREENLAND

P. 16   *"The fish industry is heartened"*   Ancel Keys, Joseph T. Anderson, and Francisco Grande, "'Essential' Fatty Acids, Degree of Unsaturation, and Effect of Corn (Maize) Oil on the Serum-Cholesterol Level in Man," *Lancet*, January 12, 1957, p. 66.

P. 18   *On the first of what*   We tend to think of Denmark as a fish-eating nation, but Denmark produces more pigs and pork products than any other country: its national snack food is the hot dog *(pølse)*. Most of

Denmark's fish are reduced to fish meal for feeding its livestock, and until recently, much of its fish oil was hydrogenated to make margarine and shortening.

P. 21   *In their paper in the* Lancet   H. O. Bang, J. Dyerberg, and Aase Brøndum Nielsen, "Plasma Lipid and Lipoprotein Pattern in Greenlandic West-Coast Eskimos," *Lancet*, June 5, 1971, pp. 1143–46; quotations, 1145. See also H. O. Bang and Jørn Dyerberg, "Plasma Lipids and Lipoproteins in Greenlandic West Coast Eskimos," *Acta Medica Scandinavica* 192 (1972): 85–94.

P. 23   *When Dyerberg and Bang separated out*   J. Dyerberg, H. O. Bang, and N. Hjørne, "Fatty Acid Composition of the Plasma Lipids in Greenland Eskimos," *American Journal of Clinical Nutrition* 28 (1975): 958–66.

THREE. HOW THE OMEGAS GOT THEIR NAME

P. 26   *But he didn't go home*   Ralph T. Holman, "Nutritional and Metabolic Interrelationships between Fatty Acids," *Federal Proceedings* 23 (1964): 1067.

P. 27   *If they are given a small amount of the right*   George O. Burr and Mildred M. Burr, "A New Deficiency Disease Produced by the Rigid Exclusion of Fat from the Diet," *Journal of Biological Chemistry* 82 (1929): 364. See also the Burrs' paper "On the Nature and Role of the Fatty Acids Essential in Nutrition," *Journal of Biological Chemistry* 86 (1930): 587–621; Ralph T. Holman, "George O. Burr and the Discovery of Essential Fatty Acids," *Journal of Nutrition* 118 (1988): 535–40; and George O. Burr, "The Essential Fatty Acids Fifty Years Ago," in *Golden Jubilee International Congress on Essential Fatty Acids and Prostaglandins*, ed. Ralph T. Holman (Oxford: Pergamon Press, 1981), xxvii–xxix.

P. 28   *Fatty acids with three double bonds*   That the Burrs mentioned linolenic acid as a possible essential fatty acid in their first papers, then dismissed it, was and remains confusing to this day. Linolenic acid is a general, or common, name for any fatty acid with three double bonds. It does not specify, nor were the Burrs able to determine with existing methods, the length of the fatty acid or the location of those double bonds. Today, it is sometimes said that the linolenic acid referred to in the Burrs' early papers was not alpha linolenic acid but two other forms of linolenic acid that belong in the omega-6 family and are the intermediaries between linoleic and arachidonic acid (gamma linolenic acid and dihomo-gamma-linolenic acid). But this can't be true, since linseed oil doesn't contain either of these two forms. Linseeds (also called *flaxseeds*), like most terrestrial plants, lack the enzyme that is necessary to add double bonds to linoleic or alpha linolenic acid—the delta-6 desaturase, as it is called.

P. 29   *The Burrs' volunteer*   William Redman Brown, Arild Edsten Hansen, George Oswald Burr, and Irvine McQuarrie, "Effects of Prolonged Use of Extremely Low-Fat Diet on an Adult Human Subject," *Journal of Nutrition* 16 (1938): 511–24.

P. 30   *The Hormel Company*   In 1938 Jay Hormel, the CEO of the company, made arrangements with the University of Minnesota to sponsor four professors in the area of food science, providing each with $25,000 a year.

P. 31   *"In contrast to all other fatty acids"*   R. Schoenheimer and D. Rittenberg, *Physiological Reviews* 20 (1940): 218.

P. 31   *The triglycerides in fish oils*   Some readers may be wondering why the seemingly simple and bland substances we call fats and oils contain so many different fatty acids. Scientists don't know, but their best guess is that this diversity prevents crystallization, the exact thing that Holman was trying to achieve. "Crystals are bad news in cells because they punch holes in things," says Robert Ackman, one of the world's foremost fish biologists. "By mixing fats up, you have much less a risk of this happening." This probably explains why fish, especially cold-water fish, have the greatest number of different fatty acids and triglycerides of any living thing. "The fatty acids in fish oil come by the dozen," Ackman goes on. "The triglycerides are in the thousands."

P. 33   *Because of the difficulty of crystallizing polyunsaturates*   Many of Holman's techniques for separating polyunsaturates are still being used today.

P. 36   *Hansen began testing babies*   Brown, Hansen, Burr, and Mc-Quarrie, "Effects of Prolonged Use of Extremely Low-Fat Diet on an Adult Human Subject."

P. 36   *Hansen and Holman were also able to show*   Ralph T. Holman, "ω3 and ω6 Essential Fatty Acid Status in Human Health and Disease," in *Handbook of Essential Fatty Acid Biology: Biochemistry, Physiology, and Behavioral Neurobiology,* ed. Shlomo Yehuda and David I. Mostofsky (Totowa, N.J.: Humana Press, 1997), 139–82. See also Ralph T. Holman, "The Slow Discovery of the Importance of ω3 Essential Fatty Acids in Human Health: Evolution of Ideas about the Nutritional Value of Dietary Fat," *Journal of Nutrition* 128, suppl. 2 (1998): 427S–433S; A. E. Hansen et al., "Essential Fatty Acids in Human Nutrition III. Clinical Manifestations of Linoleic Acid Deficiency," *Journal of Nutrition* 66 (1958): 564–70.

P. 37   *Now, he and Mohrhauer gave rats*   Fatty acids don't keep very well, so Holman and Mohrhauer actually fed their rats methyl esters of the fatty acids (linoleate, linolenate, etc.). Since the methyl esters are equivalent in most ways to fatty acids, I have avoided the added complication of these extra terms.

P. 38   *The explanation that Holman ultimately chose*   The existence of the enzymes that desaturate and elongate fatty acids (the elongases and desaturases) was at first purely hypothetical. Later, physical evidence and proof would be found for all but one of the enzymes, the one that was thought to catalyze the last step in DHA synthesis: the so-called delta-4 desaturase. The synthesis of DHA, as it turns out, is more complicated than first hypothesized. It involves a couple of extra steps and a cell organelle called the peroxisome—but no delta-4 desaturase.

P. 41   *Holman and Mohrhauer introduced*   Ralph T. Holman and Hans Mohrhauer, "A Hypothesis Involving Competitive Inhibitions in the Metabolism of Polyunsaturated Fatty Acids," *Acta Chemica Scandinavica* 179 (1963): S84n.

P. 41   *In a footnote to a paper*   Joseph J. Rahm and Ralph T. Holman, "The Relationship of Single Dietary Polyunsaturated Fatty Acids to

Fatty Acid Composition of Lipids from Subcellular Particles of Liver," *Journal of Lipid Research* 5 (1964): 169n.

FOUR. MONSIEUR CHOLESTEROL

P. 45   *That was Ancel Keys*   William Hoffman, "Meet Monsieur Cholesterol," University of Minnesota *Update*, Winter 1979, at http://mbbnet.umn.edu/hoff/hoff_ak.html (accessed October 1, 2005).

P. 46   *In the late 1950s*   "Facts on Fats," *Time*, March 30, 1959, p. 51; Ancel Keys et al., *Seven Countries: A Multivariate Analysis of Death and Coronary Heart Disease* (Cambridge, Mass.: Harvard University Press, 1980).

P. 47   *"Starved people cannot be taught"*   Hoffman, "Meet Monsieur Cholesterol."

P. 47   *But others experienced a positive benefit*   Descriptions of this wartime trend can be found in Haqvin Malmros, "The Relation of Nutrition to Health," *Acta Medica Scandinavica*, suppl. 245 (1950): 137–53; Axel Strøm and R. Adelsten Jensen, "Mortality from Circulatory Disease in Norway 1940–1954," *Lancet*, January 20, 1951, pp. 126–29; and J. O. Leibowitz, *The History of Coronary Heart Disease* (London: Wellcome Institute of the History of Medicine, 1970).

P. 48   *To be sure, some earlier reports*   I. Snapper, *Chinese Lessons to Western Medicine: A Contribution to Geographical Medicine from the Clinics of Peiping Union Medical College*, 2nd ed. (New York: Grune and Stratton, 1965), 9–31, 158, 337–79.

P. 49   *But Keys's experiments*   Ancel Keys, "Atherosclerosis: A Problem in Newer Public Health," *Journal of Mt. Sinai Hospital* 20 (1953): 125.

P. 49   *Keys researched the fat content*   Ibid., 134.

P. 50   *"buckshot hitting a page"*   This memorable analogy came from David Kritchevsky of the Wistar Institute in Philadelphia.

P. 50   *"But the selection"*   J. Yerushalmy and Herman E. Hilleboe, "Fat in the Diet and Mortality from Heart Disease," *New York State Journal of Medicine*, July 15, 1957, p. 2346.

P. 50   *At first, Keys didn't even distinguish between the effects*   A good overview of Ed Ahrens's early work and the confusion surrounding the effects of the different fatty acids is provided in his paper "Seminar on Atherosclerosis: Nutritional Factors and Serum Lipid Levels," *American Journal of Medicine* 23 (1957): 928–52. The different styles of Ahrens and Keys—cautious and reflective versus dogmatic—come out clearly in their papers, and it's worth reading papers by each to get a sense of how Keys's personality may have shaped the field.

P. 51   *"The fish industry is heartened"*   Ancel Keys, Joseph T. Anderson, and Francisco Grande, "'Essential' Fatty Acids, Degree of Unsaturation, and Effect of Corn (Maize) Oil on the Serum-Cholesterol Level in Man," *Lancet*, January 12, 1957, p. 66.

P. 52   *But the intake of saturated fats had been declining*   These data appear in *Diet and Health: Implications for Reducing Chronic Disease List* (Washington, D.C.: National Academy Press, 1989), 56; they came originally from R. M. Marston's unpublished data (United States Department of Agriculture/Human Nutrition Information Service, 1986).

FIVE. FISHY FATS

P. 54   *But on Dyerberg and Bang's second trip to Greenland*   H. O. Bang, J. Dyerberg, and N. Hjørne, "The Composition of Food Consumed by Greenland Eskimos," *Acta Medica Scandinavica* 200 (1976): 69–73; H. O. Bang, J. Dyerberg, and H. M. Sinclair, "The Composition of the Eskimo Food in North Western Greenland," *American Journal of Clinical Nutrition* 33 (1980): 2657–61.

P. 55   *In the United States*   Dr. Gio Gori, transcript of the hearings before the U.S. Senate Select Committee on Nutrition and Human Needs, *Diet Related to Killer Diseases*, 94th Cong., 2nd sess., July 28, 1976, p. 182.

P. 55   *In 1984, six years after Dyerberg*   "Lowering Blood Cholesterol to Prevent Heart Disease," *NIH Consensus Development Conference Statement* 5, no. 7 (December 10–12, 1984): 1–11; online at http://

consensus.nih.gov/cons/047/047_statement.htm (accessed October 6, 2003). See also J. Dyerberg, H. O. Bang, E. Stoffersen, S. Moncada, and J. R. Vane, "Eicosapentaenoic Acid and Prevention of Thrombosis and Atherosclerosis?" *Lancet*, July 15, 1978, pp. 117–19.

P. 57   *Keys had published a formula*   Ancel Keys, J. T. Anderson, and F. Grande, "Serum Cholesterol Response to Changes in the Diet," *Metabolism* 14 (1965): 776.

P. 57   *Bang and Dyerberg concluded*   Bang, Dyerberg, and Hjørne, "The Composition of Food Consumed by Greenland Eskimos," 72.

P. 58   *Sinclair had been interested*   H. M. Sinclair, "Deficiency of Essential Fatty Acids and Atherosclerosis, Etcetera," letters to the editor, *Lancet*, April 7, 1956, p. 381.

P. 58   *Bang and Dyerberg didn't know*   Jeannette Ewin, *Fine Wines and Fish Oil: The Life of Hugh Macdonald Sinclair* (Oxford: Oxford University Press, 2001), 40.

P. 59   *"In Hudson Bay, far far away"*   H. M. Sinclair, "The Diet of Canadian Indians and Eskimos," *Proceedings of the Nutrition Society* 12 (1953): 69.

P. 60   *They published their findings*   Sune Bergström, Henry Danielsson, and Bengt Samuelsson, "The Enzymatic Formation of Prostaglandin E2 from Arachidonic Acid," *Biochimica et Biophysica Acta* 90 (1964): 207–10; D. A. van Dorp, R. K. Beerthuis, D. H. Nugteren, and H. Vonkeman, "The Biosynthesis of Prostaglandins," *Biochimica et Biophysica Acta* 90 (1964): 204–7. See also Sune Bergström, "Prostaglandins from Bedside Observation to a Family of Drugs," in *Progress in Lipid Research*, ed. Ralph T. Holman (Oxford: Pergamon Press, 1981), 7–12; quotation, 8.

P. 60   *Prostaglandins, later to be given*   Astute readers with an interest in chemistry may be wondering why these fatty acids have been selected to play the part of these important cellular messengers. For the same reason, probably, that these fats are so susceptible to oxidation. The carbon-interrupted cis double bonds on polyunsaturated fatty acids create hydrogens that are extremely reactive—with enzymes or with oxygen. Small amounts of these fats start chain reactions that can quickly kick-start cells in one direction or another.

P. 61   *They inhibit the enzyme*   The cyclooxygenase enzyme(s) and the lipoxygenase enzyme are the two enzymes, or types of enzymes, responsible for all the many different cell messengers made from twenty-carbon fatty acids. All these messengers now have the general name of eicosanoids, but only the products of the COX enzymes are inhibited by aspirin. These include all the prostaglandins and thromboxanes, known collectively as prostanoids. The products of the lipoxygenase enzyme are known as leukotrienes and are also involved in inflammation.

P. 61   *Now, Vane was about to fill out*   S. Moncada and J.R. Vane, "Unstable Metabolites of Arachidonic Acid and Their Role in Haemostasis and Thrombosis," *British Medical Journal* 34, no. 2 (1978): 129–35.

P. 64   *The paper ended with the suggestion*   Dyerberg et al., "Eicosapentaenoic Acid and Prevention of Thrombosis and Atherosclerosis," 119.

P. 64   *A 1979 letter to the* Lancet   G. Hornstra, E. Haddeman, and F. TenHoor, "Fish Oils, Prostaglandins, and Arterial Thrombosis," *Lancet*, November 17, 1979, p. 1080. Dyerberg and Bang responded with a letter of their own: J. Dyerberg, H.O. Bang, and O. Aagaard, "α-Linolenic Acid and Eicosapentaenoic acid," *Lancet*, January 26, 1980, p. 199.

P. 65   *"An extremely frequent disorder"*   Peter Freuchen, quoted in H. O. Bang and H. Dyerberg, "The Bleeding Tendency in Greenland Eskimos," *Danish Medical Bulletin* 27, no. 4 (1980): 202.

P. 65   *They thought they had solved*   J. Dyerberg and H.O. Bang, "Haemostatic Function and Platelet Polyunsaturated Fatty Acids in Eskimos," *Lancet*, September 1, 1979, pp. 433–35.

P. 66   *Back in England, the elderly Sinclair*   There are wild cards in this field besides Hugh Sinclair, researchers who gave essential fatty acids a bad name because their enthusiasm for the benefits of a particu-

lar fat or oil went far beyond their science. David Horrobin, the articu-
late and passionate promoter of evening primrose oil—an oil rich in the
omega-6 fat gamma linolenic acid—is probably the best known. Horrobin established an institute to market and explore the medicinal uses
of evening primrose oil and even started a medical journal to promote
his ideas. When he died in 2003, Caroline Richmond ignored admoni-
tions about not speaking ill of the dead to write a very controversial obit-
uary in the *British Medical Journal* in which she declared that Horrobin
"may prove to be the greatest snake oil salesman of his age" ("Obituar-
ies: David Horrobin," *British Medical Journal* 326 [2003]: 885). Health
food stores are full of products containing evening primrose oil or
gamma linolenic acid, a source of confusion for patrons looking for
omega-3s and a testament to the lasting influence of bad science supported by a charismatic figure.

P. 66   *They have a beneficial effect*   William S. Harris, William E.
Connor, and Martha P. McMurry, "The Comparative Reductions of the
Plasma Lipids and Lipoproteins by Dietary Polyunsaturated Fats:
Salmon Oil Versus Vegetable Oils," *Metabolism* 32 (1983): 179–84.
William Connor and his colleagues had actually made the discovery that
seafood has a beneficial effect on blood lipids long before, in the 1960s,
when he gave research subjects large amounts of cholesterol-rich shell-
fish and observed that their serum cholesterol didn't rise as expected.
But he didn't understand, or publish, these findings until the Greenland
studies provided an explanation for them.

P. 66   *And DHA, . . . as the Boston physician Alexander Leaf discovered*
A. Leaf, "Omega-3 Fatty Acids and Prevention of Ventricular Fibrilla-
tion," *Prostaglandins, Leukotrines, and Essential Fatty Acids* 52 (1995):
197–98.

P. 67   *In England's Diet and Reinfarction Trial*   M.L. Burr et al.,
"Effects of Changes in Fat, Fish, and Fibre Intakes on Death and
Myocardial Reinfarction: Diet and Reinfarction Trial (DART)," *Lancet*,
September 30, 1989, pp. 757–61.

P. 67   *But Dyerberg and Bang showed*   See Bang and Dyerberg, "The
Bleeding Tendency in Greenland Eskimos," 202–5; H. O. Bang and

J. Dyerberg, "Personal Reflections on the Incidence of Ischaemic Heart Disease in Oslo during the Second World War," *Acta Medica Scandinavica* 210 (1981): 245–48.

SIX. TREE LARD AND COW OIL

P. 73   *Lecithin is a naturally occurring substance*   Harold McGee, *On Food and Cooking: The Science and Lore of the Kitchen* (New York: Scribner, 1984), 607.

SEVEN. THE CHEMIST IN THE KITCHEN

P. 76   *But Holman did not think*   Joseph J. Rahm and Ralph T. Holman, "The Relationship of Single Dietary Polyunsaturated Fatty Acids to Fatty Acid Composition of Lipids from Subcellular Particles of Liver," *Journal of Lipid Research* 5 (1964): 169–76.

P. 78   *A nontoxic fat emulsion*   Erik Vinnars and Douglas Wilmore, "History of Parenteral Nutrition," *Journal of Parenteral and Enteral Nutrition* 27 (2003): 225–31.

P. 78   *By that time it was known*   Three papers by Ralph T. Holman show the development of his ideas about essential fatty acids over four decades, from the 1950s until the late 1990s: "The Function of Essential Fatty Acids," *Särtryck ur Svensk Kemisk Tidskrift* 68, no. 5 (1956): 282–90; "The Deficiency of Essential Fatty Acids," in *Polyunsaturated Fatty Acids*, ed. Wolf-H. Kunau and Ralph T. Holman (Champaign, IL: American Oil Chemists' Society, 1977), 163–82; and "ω3 and ω6 Essential Fatty Acid Status in Human Health and Disease," in *Handbook of Essential Fatty Acid Biology: Biochemistry, Physiology, and Behavioral Neurobiology*, ed. Shlomo Yehuda and David I. Mostofsky (Totowa, N.J.: Humana Press, 1997), 139–82.

P. 79   *"The well-known differences"*   D. J. Lee, J. N. Roehm, T. C. Yu, and R. O. Sinnhube, "Effect of ω3 Fatty Acids on the Growth Rate of Rainbow Trout, *Salmo gairdneri*," *Journal of Nutrition* 92 (1967): 93.

P. 80   *Shawna Renee Strobel was a blond*   My description of Shawna's accident is based on telephone interviews with her mother, Dorena

Appleby, and with Dr. Terry Hatch. I refer to Shawna as "Shawna Strobel" throughout this book, but her last name was changed to Shaw after she was adopted by her stepfather and long before her death. Dorena Strobel became Dorena Shaw, then Dorena Appleby.

P. 82   *Holman and Hatch published*   Ralph T. Holman, Susan B. Johnson, and Terry F. Hatch, "A Case of Human Linolenic Acid Deficiency Involving Neurological Abnormalities," *American Journal of Clinical Nutrition* 35 (1982): 617–23.

P. 83   *"If I were you"*   Dale Jarvis and I spoke by telephone in October 2003.

P. 84   *This was in 1985*   Prior to 1985, fish oil—specifically, cod liver oil—had, of course, been used to treat conditions other than heart disease. In the mid–eighteenth century, the English physician Samuel Kay found that cod liver oil relieved the suffering caused by rheumatism; about the same time, it was found to be beneficial in treating night blindness, brought about, as we now know, by a deficiency of vitamin A. In the early 1900s, cod liver oil was discovered to cure another vitamin deficiency disease, rickets; it became the primary source of vitamins A and D until scientists managed to produce these vitamins synthetically. Most people preferred a tablet to the oil's fishy taste, and sales of cod liver oil dropped dramatically. The oil's widespread use in England during the Second World War deservedly gets the credit for preventing outbreaks of rickets and night blindness, but it didn't do much to add to the omega-3s in the food supply, because little care was taken to prevent the fats in the cod liver oil from going rancid. Overall, ingesting the oil might even have had a negative effect since rancid fats are the source of damaging free radicals.

EIGHT. OUT OF AFRICA . . .

P. 89   *Crawford compared the fat*   M.A. Crawford, "Fatty-Acid Ratios in Free-Living and Domestic Animals," *Lancet*, June 22, 1968, pp. 1329–33.

P. 89   *But Crawford realized*   M.A. Crawford, "Are Our Cows Killing Us?" *New Scientist*, July 4, 1968, 16–17. "The original conception of animal fat as largely short saturated and mono-unsaturated acids arose from studies on depot fat and on selected animals fed high-energy diets and artificially encouraged to deposit saturated, adipose fat. The difference between the muscle and adipose tissue in free-living animals suggests that a re-evaluation of our concept of 'animal fat' might be of value," Crawford and his colleagues at the Nuffield Institute wrote in a later paper (M. A. Crawford et al., "Muscle and Adipose Tissue Lipids of the Warthog, *Phacochoerus aethiopicus*," *International Journal of Biochemistry* 1 [1970]: 657). "Perhaps the term 'animal fat' used in connection with arterial disease should be replaced with 'domestic fat,'" Crawford suggested ("Are Our Cows Killing Us?" 17).

P. 90   *Crawford adopted this idea*   M. A. Crawford and A. J. Sinclair, "Nutritional Influences in the Evolution of Mammalian Brain," in *Lipids, Malnutrition and the Developing Brain*, ed. K. Elliot and J. Knight (Amsterdam: Elsevier, 1972), 267–92. In an interview in London in 2003, Crawford told me that he considered this work to be his greatest contribution to science.

P. 90   *Crawford's explanation*   Michael Crawford and David Marsh, *The Driving Force: Food Evolution and the Future* (New York: Harper and Row, 1989).

P. 91   *Thus the omega-3 research*   Interestingly, alpha linolenic acid does not have its own story line. In animals, this parent omega-3 fatty acid appears to have no roles other than as precursor for the longer and more desaturated DHA and eicosapentaenoic acid and as a source of energy. Animal tissues contain very little alpha linolenic acid (which is either converted into longer fatty acids or burned for energy when it is ingested) but quite a lot of linoleic acid, which is essential, in its own right, for the health of the skin. A very different state of affairs is found in plants, for which alpha linolenic acid has many functions and linoleic acid is merely the precursor of this omega-3 fat.

P. 93   *Upon autopsy, Crawford found*   R. N. Fiennes, A. J. Sinclair, and M. A. Crawford, "Essential Fatty Acid Studies in Primates: Linolenic Acid Requirements of Capuchins," *Journal of Medical Primatology* 2 (1973): 166.

P. 94   *He was disappointed*   *Dietary Fats and Oils in Human Nutrition: A Joint FAO/WHO Report* (Rome: Food and Agriculture Organization of the United Nations, 1977), FAO Library Fiche AN: 40190, p. 30.

P. 95   *It had become clear that babies*   Preterm babies are especially vulnerable to the consequences of unsupplemented formulas, because the last trimester is a time of rapid brain development and a time when the placental and cord blood is particularly enriched with long-chain fatty acids.

P. 95   *By then, there was a great deal of evidence*   This is one of the few references I make to the association between intelligence and a diet adequate in omega-3s, and readers may wonder why I do not go into the subject more thoroughly. Call me a coward, but intelligence is such a controversial, hot-button issue that I fear it may distract from the importance that omega-3s have to the entire body. Plus, and most importantly, the brain requires many nutrients in order to function properly, not just omega-3s. So any attempt to draw an association between this one nutrient and human intelligence, other than in these well-controlled infant studies, would probably generate more heat than light. That said, researchers like Norman Salem at the NIH, who has been studying the effects of a deficiency in omega-3s, have found that deficient animals have a slower rate of learning and a striking reduction in the branching of their neurons. And perhaps omega-3s can explain why the mean IQ in Japan, where people consume large amounts of vegetables, seaweed, and fish, is higher, as British researcher Richard Lynn reports, than in the United States and other Western nations. "In our view," write Crawford and his wife, Sheilagh, "if you distort and depress the availability of the lipid building blocks, you are asking for a reduction in brain size and capacity" (Michael and Sheilagh Crawford, *What We Eat Today* [London: Neville Spearman, 1972], 161). See E. E. Birch et al., "A Randomized Controlled Trial of Early Dietary Supply of Long-Chain Polyunsaturated Fatty Acids and Mental Development in Term Infants," *Developmental Medicine and Child Neurology* 43 (2000): 174–81; S. E. Carlson et al., "Visual Acuity Development in Healthy Preterm Infants: Effect of Marine-Oil Supplementation," *American*

Journal of Clinical Nutrition 58 (1993): 35–42; A. Ahmad, T. Moriguchi, and N. Salem, "Decrease in Neuron Size in Docosahexaenoic Acid-Deficient Brain," *Pediatric Neurology* 26 (2002): 210–18; and Richard Lynn, "IQ in Japan and the United States Shows a Growing Disparity," *Nature* 297 (1982): 222–23.

P. 95   *Supplemented formulas*   Here, readers may be wondering why infant formulas are supplemented with both DHA and arachidonic acid when our food supply is deficient only in DHA and other omega-3s. The short answer is that human milk contains both of these long-chain polyunsaturates (as well as smaller amounts of eicosapentaenoic and alpha linolenic acid and large amounts of linoleic acid), and babies have inadequate amounts of the enzymes necessary to make all of the long-chain fats. The longer, and much more interesting, answer has to do with a 1993 study by Susan Carlson and her colleagues at the University of Tennessee in which preterm babies whose formula was supplemented with fish oil (containing DHA and eicosapentaenoic acid but not arachidonic acid) had a reduced growth rate as compared with preterm babies on a conventional formula. Growth rate, not brain or visual development, had always been the yardstick against which formulas were measured, so Carlson's study raised an obvious red flag. Carlson found that growth was associated with the level of arachidonic acid in babies (S. E. Carlson et al., "Arachidonic Acid Status Correlates with First Year Growth in Preterm Infants," *Proceedings of the National Academy of Sciences* 90 [1993]: 1073–77; see also S. E. Carlson et al., "First Year Growth of Preterm Infants Fed Standard Compared to Marine Oil n-3 Supplemented Formula," *Lipids* 27 [1992]: 901–7). The FDA, as well as the formula companies, decided it was prudent to include in supplemented formulas DHA and arachidonic acid—but not eicosapentaenoic acid. This decision has been justified by pointing to the very low level of eicosapentaenoic acid in the brain and noting that the rationale for supplementation is brain development. But eicosapentaenoic acid *is* present in breast milk, at almost the same level as arachidonic acid. We may not know why it is there, but there is certainly some good reason—and it may have to do with how long-lived, big-brained animals, such as we humans are, are designed to grow and how eicosanoids derived from this omega-3 fatty acid compete with those derived from arachidonic acid. Interestingly, breast-fed babies have a very different pattern of weight gain than formula-fed babies and tend to weigh less at one year of age. As Michael Crawford wrote more than thirty years ago, "If a factor accelerates growth, it is claimed to be beneficial. Yet from comparative biology, it is clear that animals which grow the fastest are always the least intelligent. The cow at one year after conception can weigh the same as a human after seventeen years of growth" (Crawford and Crawford, *What We Eat Today*, 146). Our old assumptions about growth—i.e., that a faster growth rate is better, or that maximal growth equals optimal growth—are probably not correct. The most immediate and important implication of all these unresolved issues is that formulas, even supplemented formulas, may still be far from ideal and thus mothers should breast-feed their babies whenever possible.

NINE. . . . AND INTO THE MEMBRANE

P. 98   *This bet led to a 1967 sabbatical in Stockholm*   W. E. M. Lands and B. Samuelsson, "Phospholipid Precursors of Prostaglandins," *Biochimica et Biophysica Acta* 164 (1968): 426–29.

P. 99   *He later determined that it was a substrate*   William E. M. Lands, Paul R. LeTellier, Leonard H. Rome, and Jack Y. Vanderhoek, "Inhibition of Prostaglandin Biosynthesis," *Advances in the Biosciences* 9 (1972): 15–28.

P. 99   *Another discovery*   William E. M. Lands, "Stories about Acyl Chains," *Biochimica et Biophysica Acta* 1483 (2000): 1–15; quotation, 4.

P. 99   *"When they can't handle the hand"*   Lands was probably thinking of the lyric written by Yip Harburg: "When I can't fondle the hand I'm fond of, I fondle the hand at hand."

P. 100   *Diets can have the same effects*   W. E. M. Lands, "Primary Prevention in Cardiovascular Disease: Moving out of the Shadows of the Truth about Death," *Nutrition, Metabolism and Cardiovascular Diseases* 13 (2003): 154–64.

P. 101   *So Lands has spent much*   Warning: these websites—http://
efaeducation.nih.gov/sig/ods.html and http://efaeducation.nih.gov—are
complicated to use. Their message, though, is simple: eat more omega-
3s and fewer omega-6s. See also Bill Lands, "Please Don't Tell Me to Die
Faster," unpublished paper, ca. 2002; and "Some Drugs Treat What
Diets Could Prevent," paper presented at the fifth congress of the International Society for the Study of Fatty Acids and Lipids, 2002, Montreal.

TEN. WHERE HAVE ALL THE OMEGA-3s GONE?

P. 105   *These tables indicated*   Artemis P. Simopoulos, Robert R. Kifer,
and Roy E. Martin, eds., *Health Effects of Polyunsaturated Fatty Acids in
Seafoods* (Orlando, Fla.: Academic Press, 1986).

P. 105   *Hydrogenation is a technique*   William Shurtleff and Akiko
Aoyagi, "History of Soy Oil Hydrogenation and of Research on the
Safety of Hydrogenated Vegetable Oils," in *History of Soybeans and
Soyfoods Past Present and Future,* at www.thcsoydailyclub.com/SFC/
MSPproducts501.asp (accessed September 27, 2005).

P. 106   *The United States Department of Agriculture*   These data
appear in *Diet and Health: Implications for Reducing Chronic Disease List*
(Washington, D.C.: National Academy Press, 1989), 56; they came
originally from R. M. Marston's unpublished data (United States
Department of Agriculture/Human Nutrition Information Service,
1986).

P. 107   *"Processed foods and alpha linolenic acid"*   Companies that
process food seek a long shelf life, meaning a matter of months, not
weeks or days. A shelf life of several weeks is entirely possible with a high
alpha linolenic acid content, says Paul Stitt, the Wisconsin baker who
was the first person to use ground flaxseed in a commercial product.

P. 108   *"Israeli Jews may be regarded"*   Daniel Yam, Abraham Eliraz,
and Elliot M. Berry, "Diet and Disease—the Israeli Paradox: Possible
Dangers of a High Omega-6 Polyunsaturated Fatty Acid Diet," *Israel
Journal of Medical Sciences* 32 (1996): 1134–43; quotation, 1134. Israel
took shape as a nation at the same time that Keys's model of heart disease

gained prominence, and the new, nutrition-conscious country took recommendations about polyunsaturated fats very seriously. Little butter is consumed in Israel, but large quantities of soybean, corn, and safflower oil are. Given this high consumption of polyunsaturates and low consumption of animal fat and cholesterol, it's not surprising that Israelis have a mean serum cholesterol of just 210 milligrams/dl. What is surprising to many observers is their very high rate of heart disease (as well as of obesity, diabetes, and many cancers). Researchers who have been looking into this paradox have compared Israelis with other populations and have found that linoleic acid constitutes about 24 percent of the total fatty acids in the adipose tissue of Israelis, as compared to 16 percent in Americans and less than 10 percent in many northern Europeans. This translates, researchers estimate, to a linoleic acid intake of about 11 percent of calories and to a ratio of linoleic to alpha linolenic acid in the Israeli diet of about 26:1. The minimum requirement for linoleic acid is about 1 percent of calories. Most countries, including Israel, have not set an upper limit.

P. 109   *Simopoulos began by testing purslane*   A. P. Simopoulos and N. Salem, Jr., "Purslane: A Terrestrial Source of Omega-3 Fatty Acids," *New England Journal of Medicine* 315 (1986): 833.

P. 109   *Then Simopoulos tested a Greek egg*   Artemis P. Simopoulos and Norman Salem, Jr., "N-3 Fatty Acids in Eggs from Range-Fed Greek Chickens," letter to the editor, *New England Journal of Medicine* 321 (1989): 1412.

P. 111   *A number of alga and plankton species*   The ability of algae to produce long-chain omega-3 fats is being taken advantage of by Martek Biosciences, a company that raises algae in large fermenters and sells the extracted, and very pure, DHA to companies producing infant formula and other foods. This DHA is uncontaminated by mercury and PCBs and has still another big advantage over fish oils. Fish oils, as we know, are messy mixtures of many different fatty acids, including DHA and eicosapentaenoic acid. But algae tend to produce oils that are predominantly DHA *or* eicosapentaenoic acid. In the interest of full disclosure, I should mention that my husband invested $5,000 in Martek after I interviewed one of its founders, David Kyle.

P. 111   *These trout exhibited*   J. D. Castel, R. O. Sinnhuber, and D. J. Lee, "Essential Fatty Acids in the Diet of Rainbow Trout *(Salmo gairdneri)*: Growth, Feed Conversion and Some Gross Deficiency Symptoms," *Journal of Nutrition* 102 (1972): 77–86.

P. 111   *Simopoulos was one of the first*   M. A. Crawford et al., "The Food Chain for n-6 and n-3 Fatty Acids with Special Reference to Animal Products," in *Dietary ω3 and ω6 Fatty Acids: Biological Effects and Nutritional Essentiality*, ed. Claudio Galli and Artemis Simopoulos (New York: Plenum Press, 1988), 5–19.

P. 112   *Data for the United States*   P. M. Kris-Etherton et al., "Polyunsaturated Fatty Acids in the Food Chain in the United States," *American Journal of Clinical Nutrition* 71 (2000): 179S–188S.

P. 113   *A second population that is very revealing*   Ralph T. Holman, Susan B. Johnson, Douglas M. Bibus, Theo C. Okeahialem, and Peter O. Egwim, "High Omega-3 Essential Fatty Acid Status in Nigerians and Low Status in Minnesotans," *World Wide Web Journal of Biology* 2 (1996–97), www.epress.com/w3jbio/vol2/holman/holman.html (accessed March 24, 2003).

P. 114   *To be sure, 1985 . . . marked the beginning of numerous studies* J. R. Hibbeln and N. Salem, Jr., "Dietary Polyunsaturated Fatty Acids and Depression," *American Journal of Clinical Nutrition* 62 (1995): 1–9; J. R. Hibbeln, "Long-Chain Polyunsaturated Fatty Acids in Depression and Related Conditions," in *Phospholipid Spectrum Disorder in Psychiatry*, ed. Malcolm Peet, Iain Glen, and David F. Horrobin (Carnforth, Lancashire: Marius Press, 1999), 195–210; and A. L. Stoll et al., "Omega 3 Fatty Acids in Bipolar Disorder: A Preliminary Double-Blind, Placebo-Controlled Trial," *Archives of General Psychiatry* 56 (1999): 407–12. Joseph Hibbeln at the NIH and Andrew Stoll at McLean Hospital in Belmont, Massachusetts, independently began studying the effects of omega-3s on mental disorders in the late 1980s. Hibbeln was struck by the large amount of fat in brain tissue and Stoll was looking for a new way to treat bipolar patients who were resistant to existing medications; he decided to try fish oil because omega-3s "looked good on paper," he told me. From their research so far, Stoll thinks that the eicosapentaenoic acid–derived eicosanoids play the important role in helping bipolar patients; Hibbeln thinks that the membrane effects of DHA are important in preventing depression, a difference that underscores the varying functions of these fatty acids. As a point of somewhat secondary interest, Stoll, a physician, remembers his days in medical school when he heard only about arachidonic acid in the biochemistry course that covered eicosanoids. There was no mention, he says, of eicosapentaenoic acid.

It's easy to imagine how changes in the fatty acid content of nervous tissue could lead to depression and other mental disorders, especially since Joe Hibbeln and Norman Salem have found a direct relationship between serotonin levels and membrane DHA content. But not as easy to see the link between fatty acids and cancer. Leonard Sauer and Robert Dauchy at the Bassett Research Institute in Cooperstown, N.Y., who have been studying this connection since the mid-1980s, have found that dietary fat has a profound effect on their ability to implant human cancer cell lines into nude immunocompromised rats—their experimental animals and the model in which these researchers study tumor growth. In rats fed corn oil as their sole fat, implantation is easy and growth of tumors is rapid. In rats fed a diet in which the corn oil is replaced by fish oil, implantation is difficult and growth is slow, if the tumor takes at all. The same is true for all the cancer lines Sauer and Dauchy have looked at, including estrogen-sensitive and estrogen-insensitive breast cancers and liver, prostate, and head and neck cancers. The researchers have spent much of the past decade looking for the mechanism behind this astonishing and very reproducible finding. In a recent paper, they and a colleague, David Blask, who studies the inhibition of cancer growth by the neurohormone melatonin, propose that it involves proteins on the surface of cells that bind free fatty acids (so-called free fatty acid receptors). When these membrane-bound proteins grab hold of an omega-3 fatty acid (or a molecule of melatonin), they initiate a cascade of events that leads to the diminished uptake of linoleic acid, the principal energy source of the tumor cells. Melatonin, of course, is secreted by the pineal gland in darkness, so a single mechanism may play a role in the association of increasing cancer rates in Western countries with both rising light levels and changing diets. This intriguing new mechanism will be the subject of future research at the Bassett Research Institute, but it probably represents only one way that dietary fatty acids affect tumor growth. Other researchers have found that eicosanoids derived from arachidonic acid are potent breast cancer stimulants and that omega-6s reduce the vulnerability of cells to free radical attack and turn on genes that prevent cell death. Omega-3s have also been found to reduce cell adhesion, an essential requirement of cancer cells before they can metastasize. For more information on the work at the Bassett Institute, see Leonard A. Sauer, Robert T. Dauchy, and David E. Blask, "Mechanism for the Antitumor and Anticachectic Effects of n-3 Fatty Acids," *Cancer Research* 60 (2000): 5289–95, and "Polyunsaturated Fatty Acids, Melatonin, and Cancer Prevention," *Biochemical Pharmacology* 61 (2001): 1455–62. See also Sung-Hee Chang et al., "Role of Prostaglandin E$_2$-Dependent Angiogenic Switch in Cyclooxygenase 2-Induced Breast Cancer Progression," *Proceedings of the National Academy of Sciences* 101 (2004): 591–96.

P. 114   *As of their most recent revision*   See "Dietary Health Guidelines: Choose Sensibly," www.health.gov/dietaryguidelines/dga2000/document/choose.htm (accessed November 10, 2004); "Know Your Fats," www.americanheart.org/presenter.jhtml?identifier=532 (accessed November 10, 2004).

P. 115   *The Institute of Medicine   Dietary Reference Intakes for Energy, Carbohydrate, Fiber, Fat, Fatty Acids, Cholesterol, Protein, and Amino Acids (Macronutrients)*, Food and Nutrition Board, Institute of Medicine (Washington, D.C.: National Academies Press, 2005), 423. Recommendations in Sweden and Japan are mentioned in Kris-Etherton et al., "Polyunsaturated Fatty Acids in the Food Chain in the United States," 184S.

P. 116   *Reducing saturated fat*   Finland best exemplifies the benefits that come from reducing fats in the diet. In the late 1960s, Finland had the highest mortality rate from heart disease in the world—by

1971, well over 700 deaths per 100,000 people—and the highest intake of saturated fats, from a diet rich in full-fat dairy products, sausages, and canned meats. In the early 1970s, the Finnish Department of Health set out to lower the incidence of heart disease in the country by changing the dietary risk factors: Finns were encouraged to switch from lard and butter to unsaturated vegetable oils and from full-fat to low-fat dairy products, as well as to lower their salt intake and increase their consumption of fruits and vegetables. By 1997, mortality from heart disease had been cut in half—still a high rate by the standards of some countries (in Greece, it was 176 per 100,000 in 1997), but an astonishing achievement in such a short period of time.

Interestingly, the Finns were spared any negative consequences of switching to unsaturated vegetable oils because the oil they switched to was rapeseed oil, which has a high alpha linolenic acid content. This feature did not figure at all into the Finnish government's decision to promote the use of vegetable oil. Rape, a cold-adapted plant, just happens to grow well at their northern latitude, making rapeseed oil economical for the Finns to buy.

P. 118   *But this change won't lead*   Another entire book could be written about the controversies and research surrounding monounsaturates—fatty acids like oleic acid with just one double bond. Ancel Keys began by grouping monounsaturates and saturates together, but subsequent experiments and the experience of the Greeks—who consume large amounts of olive oil, the most famous of the fats that are rich in monounsaturates, yet have little heart disease—led to a reevaluation of the health effects of oleic acid, which is ubiquitous in nature and a significant part of all plant and animal fats. Once it was learned that monounsaturated fats do not raise serum cholesterol as much as do saturated fats, they were embraced by many as being the healthiest of all fats. But serum cholesterol, as we know, is only a surrogate marker for heart disease; and monounsaturated fats compete with omega-3s, though not as effectively as omega-6s do. Olive oil may well have health benefits apart from its saturation index (because of a high content of antioxidants and of compounds with anti-inflammatory effects), but the bottom line about monounsaturates is that their effect will depend very much on what else people are eating. Are they eating lots of fish and greens, as the Greeks do, and thereby providing lots of omega-3 fats for their tissues? Or are they adding these monounsaturates to a diet rich in omega-6 fats? "The Greek diet is healthy not because of its olive oil content," as one researcher told me, "but because of everything else the Greeks are eating and everything they are not eating." Oil producers today are hiding behind the reputation of olive oil and are developing seeds (rapeseeds, soy beans) and oils with a higher and higher monounsaturated content. This will certainly produce some benefits by reducing the omega-6 content of these oils (and the food supply), but consumers still need sources of omega-3s.

P. 118 *European food producers* Readers may wonder whether the new oils produced by interesterification could pose a long-term danger to humans. Probably not, since the new triglycerides in these oils are made from fatty acids that the body is familiar with. Fats and oils in foods contain thousands of different kinds of triglycerides, which the body disassembles and reassembles as needed.

ELEVEN. THE SPEED OF LIFE

P. 121 *Among these researchers is Lawrence Rudel* Aaron T. Lada, Lawrence L. Rudel, and Richard W. St. Clair, "Effects of LDL Enriched with Different Dietary Fatty Acids on Cholesterol Ester Accumulation and Turnover in THP-1 Macrophages," *Journal of Lipid Research* 44 (2003): 770–79; Joseph J. Rahm and Ralph T. Holman, "The Relationship of Single Dietary Polyunsaturated Fatty Acids to Fatty Acid Composition of Lipids from Subcellular Particles of Liver," *Journal of Lipid Research* 5 (1964): 169–76.

P. 121 *And Leonard Sauer and Robert Dauchy* Leonard A. Sauer, Robert T. Dauchy, and David E. Blask, "Mechanism for the Antitumor and Anticachectic Effects of n-3 Fatty Acids," *Cancer Research* 60 (2000): 5289–95; L. A. Sauer, R. T. Dauchy, D. E. Blask, J. A. Krause, L. K. Davidson, and E. M. Daucy, "Eicosapentaenoic Acid Suppresses Cell Proliferation in MCF-7 Human Breast Cancer Xenografts in Nude Rats via a Pertussis Toxin-Sensitive Signal Transduction Pathway," *Journal of Nutrition* 135 (2005): 2124–29.

P. 121   *And Gregory Florant*   Vanessa L. Hill and Gregory L. Florant, "The Effect of a Linseed Oil Diet on Hibernation in Yellow-Bellied Marmots *(Marmota flaviventris)*," *Physiology and Behavior* 68 (2000): 431–37.

P. 123   *These effects are the subject*   A. J. Hulbert and Paul Lewis Else, "Membranes as Possible Pacemakers of Metabolism," *Journal of Theoretical Biology* 199 (1999): 257–74.

P. 124   *Hulbert and a graduate student*   P. L. Else and A. J. Hulbert, "Comparison of the 'Mammal Machine' and the 'Reptile Machine': Energy Production," *American Journal of Physiology* 240 (1981): R3–9.

P. 126   *It is the concentration of this highly unsaturated*   This intriguing but isolated finding, that the heart rate of whales, humans, rabbits, rats, and mice goes up linearly with the amount of DHA in the heart muscle cells, was reported by the Icelandic researcher Sigmundar Gudbjarnason and his colleagues in 1978, before Hulbert and Else had begun thinking about membranes as the pacemaker of metabolism. Hulbert and Else read Gudbjarnason's paper when they were looking for mechanisms to explain their findings, and it contributed greatly to their interest in the role of fats. See Sigmundar Gudbjarnason, Barbara Doell, Gudrun Oskarsdottir, and Jonas Hallgrimsson, "Modification of Cardiac Phospholipids and Catecholamine Stress Tolerance," in *Tocopherol, Oxygen and Biomembranes: Proceedings of the International Symposium on Tocopherol, Oxygen, and Biomembranes, Held at Lake Yamanaka, Japan, September 2/3, 1977, a Naito Foundation Symposium*, ed. C. de Duve and O. Hayaishi (Amsterdam: Elsevier Scientific, 1978), 297–310.

P. 126   *The last double bond*   Hulbert and Else have not found an association between the size of an animal's brain and the DHA content of its tissues, suggesting—contrary to what Michael Crawford theorizes—that DHA is not rate limiting for brain development. Another possible constraint on brain size is an animal's ability to find glucose, the brain's preferred fuel and the building block of carbohydrates. This possibility sheds an interesting light on human evolution and behavior, particularly the universality of cooking in human societies. Cooking doesn't much change the digestibility of proteins or fats, but it does produce dramatic changes in the availability of carbohydrates to digestive enzymes: the boiling and roasting of carbohydrates results in much more glucose from a given amount of food.

P. 126   *Computer simulations and nuclear magnetic resonance studies* A. J. Hulbert, "Life, Death and Membrane Bilayers," *Journal of Experimental Biology* 206 (2003): 2308.

P. 127   *"What we see with DHA"*   Scott E. Feller, Klaus Gawrisch, and Alexander D. MacKerell, Jr., "Polyunsaturated Fatty Acids in Lipid Bilayers: Intrinsic and Environmental Contributions to Their Unique Physical Properties," *Journal of the American Chemical Society* 124 (2002): 318–26. DHA is also described as decreasing the lateral pressure on proteins, thus facilitating their changes in conformations. As the chemistry professor Erland Stevens muses in an e-mail: "Chemical reactions (whether they are performed by enzymes or not) all have to overcome an energy barrier before they occur. This barrier is called the activation energy. It exists for reactions that are favorable (exothermic) or unfavorable (endothermic). Normally, the activation energy comes from thermal energy—the kinetic motion of molecules bouncing into each other. Two molecules can collide many times without reacting. It's only when they collide with the right trajectory and sufficient energy (speed) that they will react. So, freedom of motion is very important for reactions to occur at a high rate."

P. 127   *"You couldn't be an astronaut"*   See Burton J. Litman et al., "The Role of Docosahexaenoic Acid Containing Phospholipids in Modulating G Protein-Coupled Signaling Pathways," *Journal of Molecular Neuroscience* 16 (2001): 237–42, a paper in which Litman and his colleagues suggest that DHA has the same effects on rhodopsin as it does on all the many signaling pathways that rely on similar types of protein receptors (the so-called G protein-coupled receptors).

P. 128   *Because the six double bonds*   For a general discussion of the association between high metabolic rates and short lives, see Douglas Fox, "The Speed of Life," *New Scientist*, November 1, 2003, pp. 42–45.

P. 128   *The Japanese currently*   Gina Kolata, "Some Extra Heft May Be Helpful, New Study Says," *New York Times*, April 20, 2005, A1, A22. How long the Japanese will be able to hold on to their long-lived and lean reputations will depend in part on how long they can maintain their high omega-3 intake and their low omega-6 to omega-3 ratio, one of about 4:1 in recent decades. Michihiro Sugano and Fumiko Hirahara's paper "Polyunsaturated Fatty Acids in the Food Chain in Japan," *American Journal of Clinical Nutrition* 70 (2000): 189S–196S, addresses this issue and raises concerns that "food intake varies considerably in all age groups, and only a limited number of people are consuming the recommended allowance for dietary fats" (189S).

P. 129   *Storlien was a researcher*   Leonard H. Storlien, Edward W. Kraegen, Donald J. Chisholm, Glenn L. Ford, David G. Bruce, and Wendy S. Pascoe, "Fish Oil Prevents Insulin Resistance Induced by High-Fat Feeding in Rats," *Science* 237 (1987): 885–88.

P. 129   *Storlien had already found*   L. H. Storlien et al., "Fat Feeding Causes Widespread In Vivo Insulin Resistance, Decreased Energy Expenditure, and Obesity in Rats," *American Journal of Physiology* 251 (1986): E576–E583.

P. 129   *"Not a single established case"*   H. O. Bang, J. Dyerberg, and Aase Brøndum Nielsen, "Plasma Lipid and Lipoprotein Pattern in Greenlandic West-Coast Eskimos," *Lancet*, June 5, 1971, p. 1144.

P. 131   *Storlien was searching the scientific literature*   The metabolic syndrome has been known as syndrome X since 1988, when Gerald Reaven, a researcher at Stanford University, coined the term during a lecture at the annual meeting of the American Diabetics Association.

P. 132   *Hulbert and Else looked at*   A. J. Hulbert, S. Faulks, W. A. Buttemer, and P. L. Else, "Acyl Composition of Muscle Membranes Varies with Body Size in Birds," *Journal of Experimental Biology* 205 (2002): 3561–69.

P. 132   *And the activity of one of them*   The activity of the delta-5 and delta-6 desaturases also varies between different animals, as Michael Crawford and his colleagues were the first to demonstrate. In 1975, they reported that strict carnivores show no desaturase activity at all. Strict carnivores, such as lions and carnivorous fish, cannot make DHA, eicosapentaenoic acid, or arachidonic acid out of alpha linolenic and linoleic acids. Apparently, because strict carnivores get all the long-chain polyunsaturated fatty acids they need from the animals they eat, they rely solely on the efforts of their prey rather than maintaining these enzymes, which, like all enzymes, incur some costs (J. P. W. Rivers, A. J. Sinclair, and M. Λ. Crawford, "Inability of the Cat to Desaturate Essential Fatty Acids," *Nature* 285 [1975]: 171–73).

P. 133   *The reason may well be*   About 20 to 40 percent of the human body is fat; and in adult Americans 15 to 20 percent of that fat is linoleic acid. Because this mass of omega-6 fatty acid is so large—more than 7 pounds, in some individuals—a change in dietary fats may take three years to be fully effective. See S. Dayton, S. Hashimoto, W. Dixon, and M. L. Pearce, "Composition of Lipids in Human Serum and Adipose Tissue during Prolonged Feeding of a Diet High in Unsaturated Fat," *Journal of Lipid Research* 7 (1966): 103–11.

P. 134   *Metabolism is remarkably complex*   All the effects of omega-3s really do point in the same direction: these fats are more rapidly oxidized than other fats (and thus they change the balance between oxidation and storage); they have highly beneficial effects on blood lipids; they have slightly fewer calories per gram than other fats (because their double bonds contain slightly less energy than single, saturated bonds); they produce fewer inflammatory eicosanoids (and obesity, as well as heart disease, is now thought of as having a strong inflammatory component); they reduce the expression of genes that are responsible for the body's production of fats (fatty acid synthase, for one); *and* they very strongly affect membranes, thereby changing overall metabolic rates and the behavior of individual enzymes and receptors, including the insulin receptor. Researchers other than Storlien, Hulbert, and Else have found that the substitution of fish oil for other fats in the diet of lean, healthy adults reduces body fat and increases resting metabolic rate and that the degree of obesity in human subjects is negatively correlated with the concentration of omega-3 fatty acids in abdominal fat. See C. Couet et al., "Effect of Dietary Fish Oil on Body Fat Mass and Basal Fat Oxidation in Healthy Adults," *International Journal of Obesity* 21 (1997): 637–43, and Marta Garaulet et al., "Site-Specific Differences in the Fatty Acid Composition of Abdominal Adipose Tissue in an Obese Population from a Mediterranean Area," *American Journal of Clinical Nutrition* 74 (2001): 585–91.

P. 135   *They have recently published* A. J. Hulbert, N. Turner, L. H. Storlien, and P. L. Else, "Dietary Fats and Membrane Function: Implications for Metabolism and Disease," *Biological Reviews* 80 (2005): 155–69.

P. 135   *This brings me back to Atkins* The Atkins diet is both dangerous and counterproductive for reasons having to do with the brain's preferred fuel, glucose. On a carbohydrate-restricted diet, many areas of the brain will make do with ketones, a fuel derived from fats, but some maintain their absolute dependence on glucose. In order to provide these areas with adequate amounts of this clean-burning fuel, the body breaks down not just dietary protein into its glucose and amine parts but also, if need be, the protein in muscles. This loss of muscle gives the dieter the illusion of losing weight but is self-defeating in the long run, since muscle is such a metabolically active tissue and is hard to maintain as we age. Any form of the Atkins diet that is rich in saturated and omega-6 fatty acids and short in omega-3s is also dangerous for the many reasons spelled out in this book.

P. 136   *"Good nutrition does not"* Corinne Shear Wood, *Human Sickness and Health: A Biocultural View* (Palo Alto, Calif.: Mayfield Publishing, 1979), 57.

P. 136   *How great a bargain* Robert Pear, "Health Spending Rises to 15% of Economy, a Record Level," *New York Times*, January 9, 2004, A16.

TWELVE. PUTTING OMEGA-3s BACK INTO *YOUR* FOOD SUPPLY

P. 144   *Omega-3 fatty acids have also been found* Joseph R. Hibbeln, "Seafood Consumption, the DHA Content of Mothers' Milk and Prevalence Rates of Postpartum Depression: A Cross-national, Ecological Analysis," *Journal of Affective Disorders* 69 (2002): 15–29; Sjúrdur Fródi

Olsen and Niels Jørgen Secher, "Low Consumption of Seafood in Early Pregnancy as a Risk Factor for Preterm Delivery: Prospective Cohort Study," *British Medical Journal* 324 (2002): 447–50.

THIRTEEN. THE PROOF IS IN THE PUDDING

P. 148   *Recommendations to reduce dietary cholesterol*   The role of cholesterol in brain function and the dubious wisdom of blocking cholesterol synthesis are underscored by the recent finding that people with high levels of serum cholesterol (200 mg and above) score better on a variety of tests measuring mental ability. Researchers who reported this finding, as part of the long-term Framingham Heart Study, said the link between high cholesterol and mental skills appeared clear and they are concerned that it might encourage patients to go off their cholesterol-lowering medications. One of them, Boston University's Merrill Elias, called the trade-off not worth it, asking, "Do you want to be a very intelligent person when you're talking to the person who's putting a stent in you because you have heart disease?" (quoted in Eric Nagourney, "The Smart Side of Cholesterol," *New York Times*, March 29, 2005, F9). It's only our obsession with cholesterol, though, that makes us have to choose between optimal function of brain and heart. On a diet that is high in omega-3s, both can function well.

P. 149   *In the patients who took the supplement*   "Dietary Supplementation with n-3 Polyunsaturated Fatty Acids and Vitamin E in 11,324 Patients with Myocardial Infarction: Results of the GISSI-Prevenzione Trial," *Lancet*, August 7, 1999, pp. 447–55.

P. 149   *In a prospective study within the Physicians' Health Study*   C. M. Albert et al., "Blood Levels of Long-Chain n-3 Fatty Acids and the Risk of Sudden Death," *New England Journal of Medicine* 346 (2002): 1113–18.

P. 149   *In another recent analysis*   K. He et al., "Accumulated Evidence on Fish Consumption and Coronary Heart Disease Mortality: A Meta-analysis of Cohort Studies," *Circulation* 109 (2004): 2705–11.

P. 150   *Is it, as the physician Clemens von Schacky*   W. S. Harris and C. von Schacky, "The Omega-3 Index: A New Risk Factor for Sudden

Cardiac Death," *Preventive Medicine* 39 (2004): 212–20; William S. Harris and Clemens von Schacky, "The Omega-3 Index: A New Predictor of Risk for Cardiac Mortality," *International Society for the Study of Fatty Acids and Lipids (ISSFAL) Newsletter* 11, no. 3 (2004): 3–9.

P. 151   *If you live in a state that permits direct testing*   As of October 2005, the states that permit direct testing by consumers are Alaska, Colorado, Delaware, Indiana, Kansas, Louisiana, Minnesota, Missouri, Montana, Nebraska, New Hampshire, New Mexico, Ohio, Oklahoma, South Dakota, Texas, Utah, Vermont, Virginia, West Virginia, and Wisconsin, as well as Washington, D.C.

ACKNOWLEDGMENTS

I was a visiting professor at Davidson College in North Carolina while I researched this book, so many of my acknowledgments are directed to people at that small, stellar college in the South. Erland Stevens, in particular, spent hours discussing all things chemical with me, and I hope that something of his enthusiasm for molecules comes out in these pages. Pat Peroni answered my questions about plants and botany, and Joyce Carnavalle allowed me to sit in on her class on animal nutrition. Joe Gutekanst, Jean Coates, and the rest of the library staff made that building my home away from home, and Joe was so quick at locating arcane articles that I began to think that Davidson was the hub of all interlibrary loans. Some of my students—Kathleen Tanner, Jenny Saleeby, Casey Cox, Jessica Broaddus, and Leigh Anne Hoskins—contributed original research and ideas to this book, and I hope that they, and all my students, got nearly as much out of my classes as I did.

There would have been no book to contribute to, however, without the many scientists, government officials, farmers, fishmongers, food industry spokespersons, and other individuals who patiently submitted to my repeated questioning, in person or by telephone and e-mail. They are too numerous to name individually, but I'd like to give special thanks to Doug Bibus, who made my visits with Ralph Holman possible and who gave me a hands-on demonstration of gas-liquid chromatography (using my blood for the sample); Ralph Holman, who didn't allow his failing memory to put an end to our interviews and who shared his daily repast of herring on toast; Jørn Dyerberg, for the excuse to visit his delightful town of Copenhagen and for showing me the sealskin-covered diaries in which he keeps his photographs from the trips to Greenland; Lars Hansen and his wife, for the morning at their pig farm in Hyldegaard and the candlelit breakfast; Len Storlien and Bill Lands, for all their insights and for putting up with periods of almost daily e-mails; Tony Hulbert, for the visit with the naked mole rats at CCNY; Joe DiMauro and all the other boys at Mount Kisco Seafood, who maintained good humor toward their customers, this interviewer, and their fish, even on a day when the power had gone off; and Dorena Appleby, for speaking to me about her daughter Shawna Renee Strobel. Bill Lands, Len Storlien, Erland Stevens, and Tony Hulbert also read and commented on the book when it was in manuscript form; Elizabeth Beautyman and Jim Logan brought their perspectives as physicians to it and Suzanne Ironbiter, her viewpoint as an omnivorous reader. Paul Thomas and Sharron Dalton reviewed the manuscript for the Press and made a number of excellent suggestions, and Alice Falk and Dore Brown gave it a thorough polishing. I am extremely grateful for the time and comments of all these readers, but the responsibility for any lingering errors and omissions is my own. Encouragement to write the story of this research came from Juree Sondker and Jane Lear and from my editors Darra

Goldstein and Sheila Levine, who must have wondered, sometimes, whether this book would see the light of day. The librarians at the Katonah Village Library were of enormous help (as always), as were my husband and daughters—in countless ways.

INDEX

Italicized page numbers refer to figures.

TEXT
10/14 Janson
DISPLAY
Interstate
COMPOSITOR
Sheridan Books, Inc.
INDEXER
Sharon Sweeney
ILLUSTRATOR
Dartmouth Publishing
PRINTER AND BINDER
Sheridan Books, Inc.

CALIFORNIA STUDIES IN FOOD AND CULTURE
DARRA GOLDSTEIN, EDITOR

1. *Dangerous Tastes: The Story of Spices*, by Andrew Dalby
2. *Eating Right in the Renaissance*, by Ken Albala
3. *Food Politics: How the Food Industry Influences Nutrition and Health*, by Marion Nestle
4. *Camembert: A National Myth*, by Pierre Boisard
5. *Safe Food: Bacteria, Biotechnology, and Bioterrorism*, by Marion Nestle
6. *Eating Apes*, by Dale Peterson
7. *Revolution at the Table: The Transformation of the American Diet*, by Harvey Levenstein
8. *Paradox of Plenty: A Social History of Eating in Modern America*, by Harvey Levenstein
9. *Encarnación's Kitchen: Mexican Recipes from Nineteenth-Century California: Selections from Encarnación Pinedo's* El cocinero español, by Encarnación Pinedo, edited and translated by Dan Strehl, with an essay by Victor Valle
10. *Zinfandel: A History of a Grape and Its Wine*, by Charles L. Sullivan, with a foreword by Paul Draper
11. *Tsukiji: The Fish Market at the Center of the World*, by Theodore C. Bestor
12. *Born Again Bodies: Flesh and Spirit in American Christianity*, by R. Marie Griffith
13. *Our Overweight Children: What Parents, Schools, and Communities Can Do to Control the Fatness Epidemic*, by Sharron Dalton
14. *The Art of Cooking: The First Modern Cookery Book*, by The Eminent Maestro Martino of Como, translated and annotated by Jeremy Parzen, with an introduction by Luigi Ballerini, and fifty modernized recipes by Stefania Barzini
15. *The Queen of Fats: Why Omega-3s Were Removed from the Western Diet and What We Can Do to Replace Them*, by Susan Allport
16. *Meals to Come: A History of the Future of Food*, by Warren Belasco
17. *The Spice Route: A History*, by John Keay